ATHLETE BUILDER

JIM BEEBE

Resilience
Leadership Institute

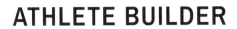

ATHLETE BUILDER

CONTENTS

PRAISE FOR ATHLETE BUILDER

"Jim Beebe's book the *Athlete Builder* delivers all the essentials to develop the mindset needed to be a highly capable individual. Great book to advance yourself in sport but also in your workplace and life in general."

-*Shane Sweatt,* Founder of the Sweatt Shop and CrossFit Conjugate

"In *Athlete Builder*, the foundation of an athlete's success lies in the power of mindset. Learn how it transforms training into a relentless pursuit of excellence, where every session is a step closer to greatness, and every challenge is an opportunity to grow stronger, both mentally and physically. With the right mental approach, training becomes purposeful, nutrition becomes fuel, and recovery becomes a strategic advantage, all coming together to forge an unbreakable spirit and unstoppable drive. I highly recommend this book for anyone trying to improve in these modalities and get to the next level in sport and in life."

-*Jeff Gum,* Founder & CEO of Sunga Life / Former Navy SEAL

"Jim's decades of experience, academic learning and coaching all came together beautifully to craft this book. His expertise, passion, and ability to simplify the winning processes and mindsets that it takes to excel at a high level make this book a masterpiece for the high achiever. Truly you will have an edge and advantage on the competition after absorbing this book."

Jesse Dale, IFBB Pro Bodybuilder. Founder of Macro Millionaire

"I have had the pleasure of working with Jim for over a decade. His resilience, attention to detail, and dedication to a goal is truly inspiring. *Athlete Builder* is a time-tested solution to helping you achieve any goal."

-*Dan Brown,* USAW National Coach / Founder of Lift Lab

"I highly recommend *Athlete Builder* by Jim Beebe, an authentic author, life coach, and trainer who truly lives by the principles he shares. Drawing from his own life experiences, Beebe provides realistic and relatable lessons, emphasizing the power of small victories in achieving bigger goals. This book offers a winning formula not only for success in the gym but also in life. It's an inspiring read for anyone looking to build sustainable habits and personal growth."

-*Craig Haggard,* Indiana State Representative, Lt. Colonel U.S. Marine Corp (RET)

"Jim Beebe has provided a blueprint for athletic success. So many times, athletes and coaches get "ideas" on training, accountability, nutrition and mental training. This is a blueprint to help develop a better athlete. This applies to those that are in educational settings and the athlete that is bettering themselves later in life. This book is a tool of learned best practices...put it into consistent use and you will be more prepared than your opponent come game time."

-*Chad Dockery,* Director of Athletics at Reitz Memorial High School, Evansville, IN. 25X State Title Winners.

"Jim' perspective and application on mindset seems to clarify decisiveness, resilience, and resourcefulness for optimal athletic performance and beyond."

-*Kenny Bigbee,* Former US Navy SEAL / Founder of Dragonfly Martial Arts & Fitness / Keynote Speaker

"The *Athlete Builder Blueprint* is just that, a blueprint for developing the mental and physical traits to succeed at a high level. Through passionate, honest, and real-life stories of overcoming challenges, Jim answers the "how's" to becoming the best athlete you can become. It gives answers while holding the reader accountable to their choices. If you're a coach looking to help your athletes, an athlete wondering how to separate yourself from your peers, or looking to level up in life, this book is for you."

-*Kyle Moran,* USA Weightlifting National Coach, Manager of Health and Fitness for Special Olympics Indiana, and the Founder of the Moran Academy

"Jim, it's clear you've put your whole heart into this. Personally, I'm a very visual learner. I really like the tables you've provided to break down strategies. And I love the Strength, Weaknesses, Opportunities, & Threats (SWOT) analysis. I thought it was very useful to see SWOT's broken out on certain topics. Great work."

-*Kristy Follmar,* Two-time Boxing Champion and Indiana Boxing Hall of Famer / Co-founder of Rock Steady Boxing

"*Athlete Builder* empowers athletes and coaches with a structured approach to achieving peak performance, emphasizing core values like integrity and discipline. It provides practical strategies for mindset, training, nutrition, and recovery, making continuous improvement manageable and effective. By focusing on small, consistent efforts, the book fosters a relentless pursuit of excellence, helping athletes and coaches make a lasting impact."

-*Rich & Jimi Airey,* Hosts of Airey Bros Radio, Ultra Athletes and Coaches.

"While I was in high school, I played multiple sports (football, basketball, track/field, and baseball), and I wouldn't have been half as successful playing them if it wasn't for Unbreakable Athletics. I was able to rack up numerous accolades (all-state, all-conference, all-city) due to the unparalleled training at Unbreakable. Now as a cadet at the United States Military Academy (USMA), being physically fit is of the utmost importance. Before attending USMA, I was training consistently at Unbreakable with some of the best athletes on the west side of Indianapolis. There was no other place that set the foundation for physical excellence, structure, and discipline. I was always pushed by whoever was training me, and after every workout session I always felt that I bettered myself for having gone. I learned what hard work is like and it forced me to mature quickly; everything is earned not given. Having experienced what training in the military is like, I am so grateful to have the opportunity to train at a gym that holds you to such a high standard. Jim Beebe has been extremely flexible with training and has been able to do remote training. Because of that I am still able to pursue excellence, currently holding a near perfect (598/600) on the Army Combat Fitness Test."

-Timmy G., United States Military Academy, fourth year cadet.

"If you want to be at your peak performance by the time you are in high school or college, starting early is essential. Unbreakable Athletics and Jim Beebe help athletes find discipline and work hard. My favorite activities from Unbreakable are training with other athletes, who will push you to be better every day, and meeting new teammates that will hold you accountable."

-Hunter H., Baseball catcher for DePauw University

"My favorite thing about my time training at Unbreakable Athletics and Jim Beebe was the culture and camaraderie of our community, from the staff and coaches to the athletes and members. I love how the coaches educate the athletes and teach the reason and importance of specific movements that carry over into their sport."

-Danny N., D1 Football player for Colgate University

"Training at Unbreakable Athletics with Jim Beebe has changed my life for the better in several ways. The competitive nature and need to get better is evident in the people who walk in there every day. I can confidently say that I wouldn't be the same athlete I am without working with him and his team."

-Jack B., D1 Football player for Ball State University

"If you know Jim, you know his passion and genuine care for athlete development. He is an exceptional coach who takes a holistic approach in developing the total athlete. His knowledge in developing both the mind and body has not only allowed numerous athletes to prosper in their given sport and overall training goals, but in life as well."

-Dan Wenger, Director of Strength & Conditioning Ball State University Football

"I have been an avid reader since the 4th grade. Early on I fell in love with reading about training and its many aspects. I chased that in my academic life as well as my vocation as a sports performance coach. I have read all the greats and frankly while they deliver the knowledge I found most dry and boring. *The Blueprint for Building Champion Athletes* is not only informative it is also entertaining. If you are serious about becoming a champion athlete or training champions, I highly suggest you get a copy. IT IS WORTH IT!"

-Chad Coy, Master Coach with the Parisi Speed School and Pro Strongman

This is for all those who told me "no" and for anyone who's ever heard it before too. This book is how you say, "Oh yeah, watch me."

FOREWORD

By Zane Fakes

Strength & Conditioning Assistant, Indianapolis Colts, All-Mac and Academic All-American, Ball State University Football

This book is exactly what the title says it is. It leaves no stone unturned regarding a comprehensive approach to becoming a champion. As I was reading through it, I realized how fortunate I was to have parents that instilled many of the ideas in this book. The main point of this blueprint is that there is no substitute for hard work. Anyone can read as many books as possible about how to become successful in various ventures, but without putting the content into action, it is useless. I appreciate Jim for putting his knowledge into a book for everyone to learn. He is not afraid to give away his secrets. I believe this is because he knows his worth and that no one can execute his plan better than he can. Jim is a confident man that is relentless in his pursuit of "getting better". If someone reads this book, and puts it into practice, I have no doubt that they will accomplish whatever it is they aimed to do.

I also want to thank Jim for giving me a chance to get my start in the strength and conditioning profession. I believe he helped me look at things differently. He had a perspective that many people I associated with did not have. At the end of the day, we were more similar than different. Jim "accused" me of being too harsh on the athletes I was training at one point. But once I explained my thought process, he actually agreed with me. I hold myself to a high standard of work ethic and accountability. When I am working with someone, I expect that same commitment. In the instances that I feel the athlete has not met my expectations, I do not take that lightly. It all boils down to a few of my favorite quotes. "Nobody cares, work harder" "It takes what it takes". That is what this book lays out for the reader, a step by step approach to becoming the best.

INTRODUCTION

At the end of the day, I believe. I swallowed the "American Dream" Kool-Aid at an early age and have believed in it ever since. I'm the guy who bets on Rocky winning the big fight and the little guy going from rags to riches. I've lived this approach my entire life, for good and for bad. I'm also in my late forties now, and I have too many lessons to count in my mental databank. And yet, I'm still a believer.

I own and run Unbreakable Athletics Academy in Plainfield, Indiana. My mission in life is to make an impact on my family first and then everyone else mentally and physically. My mission statement is this: I am forging Unbreakable athletes. That means mind, body, and spirit. I've come to know that it takes more than you've ever considered at this point. It's true for you, me, or anyone else trying to maximize potential. If you're reading this book, you'll see and learn the necessary lessons to work toward your dreams. They are lessons I've learned and watched others learn; I've been on the receiving end and giving end. And they are requirements for advancement. You will have an exhaustive and Relentless approach detailed for you in your hands. Use this as a manual for referencing every year. There is no destination. There is the journey and the way. In the end, you will have in your hands an amazing, comprehensive process for becoming an Unbreakable Athlete.

There are beliefs I must impress upon you before we advance.

Each section and chapter will have tests, lessons, examples, and points that I'm making to teach you something. Everything works, and nothing works. You must explore the different ideas for yourself. Once you find one that works for you, then you must exploit that idea. You exploit by doing. I teach. You learn. Then you do, evaluate, adjust, and do again.

Here is an example for Training. Let's take a basic movement and see how overwhelmed we can get and kill our progress before we even start. Let's look at squatting. I could instruct you to build your squat to help you as an athlete. From here more questions naturally arise:

- Am I building my squat for absolute strength?
- Am I building my squat to impact my speed?
- Am I building my squat to increase my size and mass?
- Am I building my squat to impact my muscle endurance?
- Is it all of the above?

Then more questions arise:

- Which squat do I use? Back squat, front squat, overhead squat, box squat, pause squat?
- Which stance do I use to squat? Narrow, sumo, neutral, toes pointed forward, toes pointed out?
- There are a lot of bars; which do I use? Straight bar, cambered bar, buffalo bar, earthquake bar, power bar, or Olympic bar?
- How do I add resistance? Just use plates on the bar, add chains, add bands?
- What is the tempo like? Pause squats, tempo squats, speed squats, box squats, jumping squats?
- How heavy? Maximum load, sub-maximum load, for warming up, laddering up, back down sets?

- How often? Once per week, twice, three times, heavy one day, light the next?
- How does this impact next week, next month, the in-season training, offseason training?

It's overwhelming. . . seemingly. No, the intro is *not* about squatting. Here is the point: I am going to give you more good ideas than you can imagine. In fact, you won't be able to implement them all. You shouldn't. Please don't. But for each topic, write them down. Have them in a place and save them. Then pick one or at most two ideas in a section and implement them. Work on those habits for two weeks and see the effects. Then adjust. Maybe you keep at it, maybe you evolve the idea, or maybe you pivot to a different but similar idea. Either way, do *not* implement all the ideas. Just like you wouldn't implement every squat variation I listed, just pick one or two and execute. Execute Relentlessly.

Go all in. Whatever you think "all in" is, you're wrong. It's much more than that. I believe in the "emotion creates motion" mantra you hear from others like Tony Robbins. I do motivational speaking, mindset training for athletes. Each speaking event we start with one set of push-ups. I say, "Get in at least a good set of twenty-five push-ups." Then we do one set together. I like to give the test first, then the lesson. I'll see awesome push-ups, crap push-ups, some done on their knees but absolutely to the best of their ability and some on their toes that are embarrassing. Then I ask for a show of hands, "Who almost got twenty-five? Who hit twenty-five? Thirty? Thirty-five? Forty? Forty-five? Fifty?" After fifty, I ask, "Okay. How many did you get?" My guy Lucas Lorian, a strength and conditioning coach, simply stopped in the mid sixties when I was speaking to his Northside High School football team in Fort Wayne, Indiana. The test is telling. Who does the push-ups with Integrity? Who is strong, and who is weak? Who can't do the required work? Who does the minimums? (Very important insight.) Who goes beyond? Who goes beyond and to the point of failure? Who goes beyond and takes the David Goggins approach of "taking souls," reaching such a high level of performance that the opponent mentally gives up? Whose mindset in the group is to go so far that you know you have no chance ever of beating him at anything? If you're going to do something, go all in. See it all the way through. And smash it. If you're trying to get to the Statue level (more on that later), then anything but "all in" won't even come close to getting you there.

Louie Simmons ran the best powerlifting gym in the world at West-Side Barbell (WSBB) in Columbus, Ohio. It's still around today. WSBB is legendary. Louie put out so much of his knowledge in books, videos, seminars, and in-person visits to his gym. He was always asked, "How can you divulge all your secrets? How can you tell athletes and competitors what you're doing? Aren't you worried they will take your information and beat you?"

"Easy," Louie replied. "Almost no one will ever do it. They won't do all the necessary work to win. They'll quit because it's hard."

That's the deal too. Some of you will read this book, think it has good ideas, and let it gather dust on the shelf. It's a manual. Keep coming back to it. Write in it. Mark it up. But do the work. Execution is what matters. It's everything. If you find three things you love and they make a difference for you, then Just Do It (Nike)! Stop reading. Go out and do the work. Get better. If you plateau, come back to the book and look up what to do next. Then Just Do It! The point is to work. Work like this is your only shot. And take the "max push-ups" approach.

Lastly, here's a little more about me. I'm well above average and great at some things and pathetically terrible at others. I'll provide examples throughout the book to illustrate. I'm good at suffering. I'm quite analytical. I read people well. I'm painfully authentic and honest. I have very little fear, and what I do have, I just walk through. On the other side, I am moderately athletic, struggle painfully to focus, have little to no empathy, speak too quickly or even stutter, and I have a quick temper which I must "breathe my way through." My approach is simply to keep going until I reach my next target. Then I assess, adjust, and repeat the approach for my next target from now until I pass away.

I grew up like most people. I had a ton of bad breaks and crap dealt to me. And I also had a lot of awesome, fortunate breaks. We had very little money but were wealthy by a lot of other standards. I've had huge wins and had much larger losses in my life, personally and professionally. At times, my decisions have been amazing, cunning, profitable, and out of nowhere. And the next day, I've been so painfully wrong I wonder what I am doing with my life. I've been entrepreneurial my entire life from a young age. I've been working with and training athletes the last ten-plus years. I barely graduated with a business degree from Purdue University in 1997. Then in 2009 I was at the top of my class in the master of finance program also at Purdue.

I read daily. I read books by pro athletes, Navy SEALs, business leaders, philosophers, motivational speakers. When I'm not reading, I'm listening to podcasts or watching videos. I put it all together for my business at Unbreakable Athletics. Once their careers are over, pro athletes author books about their lessons and how you can apply them to life. So do the military leaders. The theory is that A leads to B. Football lessons lead to life lessons. Military habits lead to life habits. If that's true, then the opposite is also true. B can lead to A. Life lessons can lead to football or tennis lessons. Life habits can be examples for military habits. That's what you have here. You'll have business lessons, athletic lessons, philosophical lessons, and science lessons compiled for you so you can apply the different ideas to win at sports. In any arena, your plays, games, seasons, and championships will come down to Inches. Small, minute details, habits, and executions will determine winning and losing, life and death. Results are all that matter then. Your Inches add up. Inches accumulated Relentlessly lead to greatness. This book is your process for greatness.

Book Layout

The first part of the book is about you and your identity. We must explore some ideas and reasons why you're actually here. We must uncover and identify your identity and purpose for competing in sports. In addition, we must set the standards for how we do things. There must be critical components that guide us and dictate our actions. These overarching principles supply the fuel for doing the necessary work. We preach six Core Values throughout this book, at my gym, and when working with athletes: Integrity, Discipline, Kaizen, Teamwork, Enjoyment, and Sisu. The word we use to apply each principle is, Relentless. We will dive deeper into this area and more in later chapters. The point is that as we do more work and accomplish more tasks, we improve our success in the sports arena.

From your Core Values, we move on to Inch Blocks, the building blocks for success. Sports are games of inches. Every inch matters and directly impacts winning and losing. Field goals in football either make it or miss by inches. A bat smashes or misses a baseball by inches. Races at all levels are won by inches or fractions of seconds. Cumulatively, everything matters. Consequently, everything matters in preparation as well. Metaphorically, I maintain that building each of the six critical components requires an additional inch for each side. One side of a block has four lines and four corners, each an inch long. Making a 3D version requires eight more inches. Stacking another block on top of the original requires more inches still. The goal is to keep building more blocks and stacking them on top of each other, thus illustrating the athlete's progression in one of the areas (in this case, Knowledge). The athlete must do the same thing for the other five areas. The more Relentlessly you build your blocks, the more likely you are to win.

The second part of the book deals with the Inch Blocks associated with your head. The first part is your Mindset. Your Mindset guides your actions and keeps you moving forward. The second part in your head is your Knowledge. Knowledge in this context pertains to the expertise required to play your sport at the highest level you can. It also pertains to the Knowledge required off the field that is also necessary for high-level athletic performance. The third and final Inch Block with your head is Teammates. Teammates is the section dedicated to improving how you perform and interact with different people. Those people include your actual teammates on the court or field, your leadership Teammates (coaches, staff, etc.), and your support Teammates (support staff, family, friends, etc.).

The third part of the book deals with your body and the Inch Blocks associated with it. First, we will explore Training your body to perform at its highest level as an athlete. Next, we will cover what fuels your body in the Nutrition section. Finally, we will work on how you can bounce back and train the next day in the Recovery section.

The fourth and final part of the book brings everything together. It will outline and systemize the processes for improving the Inch Blocks for becoming an Unbreakable Athlete. There will be assessments and feedback. Then there will be the method for constructing a plan and breaking it down annually, quarterly, monthly, daily, and weekly. At that point you will know what to do each day. And as importantly, you will know how to quickly adjust and evolve what you're doing to maximize your performance. If you improve the different Inches in your life consistently each day, then you must improve as an athlete. And anyone dedicated to doing that daily will learn the different requirements and processes to improve daily in life. We're only here for a short while, a blink in time really. We don't have time to wait. We must move forward today. Relentlessly.

CHAPTER 1

SEVEN LEVELS OF WHY

Writing and talking about lessons is great. But witnessing and seeing a lesson is better. Of course, living the lesson is best. So do yourself a favor and look up Steiner's story on YouTube when you're done reading about him. Let's discuss the German Matthias Steiner. He competed at the 2008 Olympics in Beijing in Weightlifting. Here you will see a man live out his "Why" on stage at the highest level.

First, what is weightlifting? The sport has two lifts. The first lift is the snatch. A valid snatch occurs when someone takes a barbell from the floor and moves it in one singular motion from the floor to directly overhead. He then stands up with the barbell still securely locked out overhead. His legs, arms, and hips are securely locked out. He has three attempts to lift the most he can successfully within the standards. The second lift is the clean and jerk. Like the snatch, the athlete starts with the barbell on the floor and picks it up. However, unlike the snatch, this is a two-part lift. He picks the barbell off the floor and moves it directly up to his front rack, or on top of his shoulders. Then he stands up with the weight. Finally, he must jerk the weight from his front rack up and overhead successfully. The weight is secure over his head; he's standing tall with his arms, legs, and hips locked out. Again, he has three attempts to lift the most he can. Combining the heaviest weight he lifted from each lift will result in his total. The person with the highest total in his weight class is the overall winner.

In Beijing, Steiner was in the 105 kg+ weight class. It's for the "big boys." 105+ kilograms is 231 pounds and up. After finishing his three snatches and the first two of three clean and jerks, Steiner was sitting in third place, bronze territory. And he was last to lift in his class. His next lift would be his final lift of his weight class and the entire Olympics in weightlifting.

Before we get there, let's back up a little. The year prior, 2007, Steiner was training for the 2008 Olympics, and his wife was studying for her degree. They were both young and had their lives in front of them. One day, it all changed. His wife died in a fatal car accident. Obviously, it was a huge setback. Devastating. A collapse. Then at some point, he had a choice. He could pack it in, move on, choose a different path. Or he could continue along his original path to become an Olympic champion.

The original "Olympic champion" path would be different, of course, from before the accident occurred. There was tremendous pain and loss now. But there was also increased resolve. There was increased focus. There had appeared a new and overwhelming "Why" to push and pull Steiner along. This "Why" was no longer just from him and about him. It superseded him. It was beyond himself. It was now in honor of his late wife and marriage to her. That level of force is fierce. Vicious. Singularly focused. Relentless. Unbreakable.

Fast forward to the Beijing Games. Steiner continued his journey to prepare and compete at the event. It was the day for weightlifting at the Games. It was his turn. Earlier that day, a fellow German unexpectedly won the triathlon as a significant underdog. And Steiner took that as a positive sign. Well, there are no signs. There are occurrences. All that matters is how he or you interpret the occurrence. He thought it was a good thing; therefore it was.

The snatch was first. He opened at 198 kg (435.6 lb.) for his first lift. This was only 3 kg below his all-time best of 201 kg, his personal record (PR). He started at 98.5 percent of his best lift. Obviously, margins are slim at the top. He made this lift and 203 kg (446.6 lb.) for his second attempt. His third and last attempt was a miss at 207 kg (455.4 lb.). He finished with 203 kg. It was a solid start for Steiner.

The time to transition from the snatch to the clean and jerk is not long. Mentally, the two lifts are completely different. The snatch is described as "ballet," graceful and elegant, whereas the clean and jerk is described as "MMA," an all-out, vicious fight. In warming up for the clean and jerk, Steiner started a bit "off" mentally. He was missing warm-up lifts, shaking his confidence. He missed 235 kg (517 lb.) in warm-ups and then it was his time to go for his first attempt. The coach called for his opener of 246 kg (541.2 lb.). He cleaned it up easily. However, his jerk wasn't solid, and he did not lock it out overhead, resulting in no lift. Once an attempt ends, a coach has thirty seconds before he must pick the next weight attempt. The next attempt must be at least the same weight amount or more. It can never be less. Steiner's coach selected 248 kg (545.6 lb.).

Steiner isn't happy. He isn't confident with this next amount. His focus shifts. He thinks about his misses at 235 kg in warm-ups and again at 246 kg. Now, it's an even heavier weight. The great speaker Tony Robbins always says, "Where focus goes, your energy flows." Steiner's focus and energy have been flowing down the path of destruction and failure. Fortunately, his coach steps in and makes a single observation. He points out that Steiner barely missed his last attempt. And if he hits the next one, then he will solidify a medal for himself, his country, and his wife. Steiner's focus shifts. His energy shifts. His resolve improves.

He hits his second lift. He's sitting in bronze. Good.

Most every weightlifter sits in the warm-up area in Mindset war with himself and others around him. They listen to music, either to calm themselves or pump them up. Constant "death stares" permeate the atmosphere. It's you versus a massive, obscene amount of weight. Injury risk is high. Results are on the line. There is a constant, unending pressure—internal, family, and country—everywhere. Steiner manages it differently. He listens to no music or words. He is 100 percent present and immersed in it. He absorbs everything, all the stares, all the sounds of men dropping a quarter ton of weight from overhead, all the cheers and jeers. It's overwhelming, and he simply sucks it all in and develops this level of aggression as if he were entering the gladiator arena.

Currently, his combined total is 451 kg before his final attempt. The Russian in first place sits at 460 kg after going 210 kg + 250 kg. Steiner was the last to go and needed ten more kilos. That was 10 kg (22 lb.) more than he had ever tried in his life. Ever. His coach made the call: Two hundred forty-eight kilograms to go for the win. The win would be by one single kilogram.

Steiner approached the bar in a stalking manner. He looked angry, annoyed that it was in his way. He had gone into what Tim Grover would call his "dark side" and was prepared to fight to the end. He grabbed hold of the bar, cleaned it up and caught it beautifully deep in his squat, and stood easily. Now came the fight. He gathered himself, readjusted his hands, and jerked that massive weight up and overhead. His arms were shaking as he struggled to bring his feet together to complete the lift. He did that and was still shaking. He had to show control for a "good lift" to count. Steiner later recounted that as he was doing this, he was starting to black out, his vision narrowing and darkening. In that instant, he focused and strained to tighten up and show control. He received his down command from the judges and dropped the weight. He earns three white lights, the sign of a good lift.

He was overcome. He dropped to his knees, sobbing and screaming. He clutched his face as emotion poured out. He jumped up, pulled down the straps of his singlet, revealing his shirt beneath and his crest. His thoughts pour back to his wife and their commitment and bond. The weight was lifted, physically and metaphorically. He had succeeded and met his goal, honoring himself, his wife, and his country. Later, on the podium, he was holding his gold medal and pulled out a picture of his wife. He said he didn't want to be up there alone. He wasn't. She was with him, and he won.

That is what it looks like to have a "Why" that carries you to victory. Yes, he had his own personal "Whys" for competing. But the added

"Why" from his wife's passing was beyond him. It superseded everything. It compelled him to train, prepare, and win at the highest level. It became an unstoppable power for him, and he used it to win. You can too.

Now, what about you? Here is a personal example: Every time a new prospective athlete enters Unbreakable Athletics Academy, there is a process. We start off with a brief tour and idle chit chat and pleasantries. We look around the place, and I let him or her take it all in. Then we make our way back to my office, sit down, and start. I always start with the same question. It's my favorite:

Why are you here?

For you, it's the same thing. Hopefully, you've looked around the book, read the front and back, and read the forward and intro. You sit down and sit back, and now I ask:

Why did you buy this book? Why are you here?

So, play along here as if you entered my gym, and ask yourself why you are here. Invariably I receive the same type of answers. For the adults, it's "I want to lose weight," or it's "I want to get stronger." But usually, it's to lose weight. For student athletes, it's either "I want to get stronger," or it's "I want to get faster." Truthfully, I don't care at all what your "Why" is. Zero. None. I only care that you have a "Why." And I care whether it's a strong "Why" or not. Then we can start. With a strong enough "Why," you can manage any "how." You supply the "Why." This book teaches the "how."

My gym has no air conditioning, very typical of a CrossFit, powerlifting, strongman, or sports performance gym. It hits 100+ degrees easily in the summer. People still come. It's miserable there, hot and humid. People still come. In fact, it's full. For some, it wouldn't matter what the conditions were like; they'd still show up and train. For others, the conditions could be perfect, and they'd never train. Think I'm crazy? In 2018, I went to the local fire department and police department and offered them three full months of free training at the end of the year. It was a Christmas gift to the departments thanking them for their service. Then starting January 1 of 2019, they would have to pay if they wanted to continue. Unfortunately, we only had one person take us up on it. And he quit the first of the year. Meanwhile, we had a dozen police officers and firefighters from the major city (Indianapolis) next to our suburb paying full price for years. If people want to train, they will. If they don't, there is no chance it will happen.

Back to the original question: Why are you here? Or why did you buy this book? Write down your answer.

Here is an authentic example from early in 2022. I'd never had this type of athlete enter my gym before. Brian, an eighth grader, and his family walked in, took the tour, and sat down. I asked him why he was here, and this is how it went:

Brian said, "I need to get stronger."

"Why?"

"Uh, well, I play a large instrument in the marching band, and it's heavy. I must hold it ten to twelve hours per day sometimes in the summer during practices."

I was thinking, *Ten to twelve hours per day? That sounds harder than any sport or activity that I ever played. I'm glad I didn't have to do that.* Then, I simply asked, "Why?"

"Well, the practices are hard, and currently I can't hold it long enough to keep up with the high school band."

"Why is that important? You're in eighth grade. Why does that matter to you?"

"There is the camp that lasts the entire summer in Pennsylvania," Brian answered. "I leave here soon for it and won't return until right before classes start in the fall. It's for high schoolers only. The camp invited me as an eighth grader."

Again, I thought, *That sounds infinitely harder than any sport I ever played. But I wouldn't mind traveling away from my family for the summer and having fun with a new set of friends.* Then, I simply asked again, "Why is that important to you? Why is doing well at this camp important to you?"

"We compete against other groups from around the country. There is so much on the line. We could win a national title, and I could do it as an eighth grader. There's money on the line too. And there will be college recruiters at the big events."

I had no idea of the size and scope of such an endeavor. Who knew marching bands could be so physically demanding, have money riding on it, and require so much? But greatness in any endeavor requires a deep level of commitment and execution. Then I simply asked again, "Why? Obviously, the money is great. And having college recruiters look at you is great. But why is that important to you?"

Brian had to think a bit longer for this last one. And each successive step after the first took a bit longer as well. At first, it's so easy to state the obvious, what's right in front of one's face. But deeper thought and meaning naturally requires more work. This was no different. Then he finally said, "Well, I want to play at Ohio State in their band. They are world-renowned. And we live in Indiana, so out of state tuition is too much for my family to pay. So, if I can earn a scholarship, then I can go where I want and do what I want. And my family won't have to pay for it."

And then, I said, "That's your 'why.'" Now, in this instance I only had to ask it six times. Usually, it takes between five and nine times before we can arrive at the root cause of the issue. Often it takes seven, but this time it was six. Who knows how many it will take for you? But you'll know it when you see it. And you'll really know it when you "feel" it. Invariably, it's never the first one or the first few for that matter. No one walks in and drops an emotional bomb on you with the first things out of his mouth. So, a good coach must pull it out. And an athlete must look deeply inward to understand himself. Last, write down all your "whys." The small ones are powerful too. But note them all and use them all. The pain will be easier later when you have many reasons to continue.

Temet nosce is Latin for "know thyself." There are many critical steps along the way of your journey. This first one, knowing yourself, is as critical as any step. It will point you in the right direction and give you a solid chance for success. It will function as the reminder for when setbacks occur. It will stare you in the face when you don't feel like suffering and enduring the physical and mental trauma necessary for advancement. If you have a strong, dominating "why," you can withstand any "how."

Process

Time to work. Insert cliché here. I do it all the time. "Goals without a plan are just dreams." Or "Failing to plan is planning to fail." For me, plans are good, not great. First, understand that plans are necessary, but still, they are not great. I like a SEAL mantra: A good plan today is better than a perfect plan tomorrow. Meaning, make any kind of plan, and make it decent. But get to work! Don't wait until it's refined tomorrow. By then, I would already have worked on my first plan, made one or two evolutions and iterations, and I'm already steaming ahead of you. I win. You lose. My process ends up being better because I'm faster and I adjust quicker. Inch. You must learn to do the same thing.

Process. Here's a task: In a minute, stop reading. You'll need to write things down in a journal, binder, and a planner.

Go through the 7 Steps of Why. Take your time and think deeply. Meditate if you can. Why are you here? Think broadly first and write down the first thoughts you had when you were considering this book. Then ask yourself "Why?" again and again. Get to the root cause. It's perfectly fine if there is more than one "Why." Often there are several that align. Leverage all of them. Revert to all of them for increased strength and resolve. Keep them visible in many spaces. Considering taking it easy? Read them again. Having a bad morning or a difficult day? Read them again. Know them by heart. Immerse them into your subconscious and let them take root in your identity. You are now no longer an athlete. You are an athlete with purpose, with focus. You are an athlete that is a doer. Envision the samurai warrior who is constantly on his path, called The Way. That is you, an athlete/warrior on your path to reach your perceived potential and move 10 levels beyond it. It will be scary once you see how far beyond your expectations you can travel. It will be scary once you understand what it will take. And others will find you scary seeing your Mindset, your execution, and your results. Then keep stepping forward every day. Keep building your Inch Blocks.

Here is a personal example. At age thirty-eight, I left the world of banking, finance, and investments. I had my undergraduate degree and MBA from Purdue University. I worked in finance my entire life. I was a trader for a local hedge fund. I headed up the financial investigations section for the Indiana Gaming Commission. I worked in the private bank for JP Morgan, where the minimum to invest with my team was $5 million. But that part of my life was over.

I decided it was time to make a change, and I no longer wanted to make the wealthy even wealthier. I wanted to affect people with their physical health, fitness, strength, performance, and mindset. My Cross-Fit gym opened in March of 2013 as CrossFit Unbreakable. A couple of years into it, I personally gravitated toward powerlifting and strongman. One of my coaches, Dustin Burford, started teaching me and helping me evolve at getting even stronger. CrossFit is great for being a healthy, well-rounded person. In fact, it's fantastic, and that was what we were doing for our adult athletes. For me personally, I wanted to be singularly focused and simply get bigger and stronger. That's what I did.

Fast forward to 2020. I had been lifting with that goal in mind since 2014: Just get stronger. I competed in local amateur events in the super heavyweight class. My weight reached 319 lb. as I stood six-foot-three. I could squat and deadlift six hundred pounds. I could carry three hundred pounds per hand for twenty-five feet. I could carry 750 lb. on my back and walk. Well into my forties, I could hold my own in the "old man" groups for the heavyweights.

Competing is not healthy. No one has ever said it is. It is not. Know that. Understand that. I didn't care. I was moving forward. You are too.

Now, at some point we are all told we can no longer play the game we want to play. It will happen. It happened to me. It'll happen to you. In January of 2020, I carried 305 lb. per hand in preparation for a competition in Kentucky three weeks later. I finished the lift and felt a snap in my foot. Stress fracture. Out sixteen weeks, walking in a boot. I finished rehab and got back to training. I did not realize that four months in a boot affected my gait, my hips, back, etc. I was out of alignment. That would have been okay if, and only if, I recognized it and fixed it. I didn't. A couple of months into training, I was squatting. 405 lb. was on my back for speed reps when I felt a pop and pain on the left side of my low back. This had happened before. I knew the disc was bulging in my back. I just hoped it wasn't ruptured. In the middle of the night, it took me over thirty minutes to get out of bed, to the bathroom, and return. A total nightmare. Well, long story short (or getting longer), spinal surgery was the recommendation. But my fantastic chiropractor, Dr. Josh Healy, fixed me up. I rehabbed it again and planned to start getting back after it.

My 2020 was shot. So, I started back up and looked forward to 2021. The night of the Super Bowl (early February), I was out with my wife. I had been noticing various amounts of swelling, pain, and discomfort in my left calf. My wife is a nurse, so I didn't want to tell her. I didn't want to deal with another setback. I wanted to keep going full steam ahead. I wondered if it was a blood clot, and finally that night I told her about it.

She was "thrilled" I kept that to myself. Well, the next morning we went right to the emergency room. Yup. Sure enough, blood clot. Damn it! Three more months, rehab, meds, tests, and blah blah blah. The rest of my body is squared away. But the clot means I'll always take blood-thinners the rest of my life. Now there is a threat that when I strain under weight, blood could leak out of veins and arteries, namely in the brain. That means death. In the span of fifteen months, my body said, "It's over. Find a new path."

Six months went by. I didn't lose my basic discipline. I kept training four days per week. It was just different, not as heavy, not as fun. But consistently training is part of me and my identity. I don't quit. I am not a quitter. I'm no pussy. But I couldn't train how I wanted. Finally, I sat down one day and talked to one of my coaches, Eric Farly. He's a great guy, and coach. I talked with my wife another day. I saw a bunch of doctors and got a bunch of data. I took in everything, and over the course of several days, I had a collective sit-down with myself to figure out a path. Here it was in a nutshell:

- Strongman and powerlifting were over.
- I was forty-five years old.
- I weighed 319 lb. Even with 220 lb. of muscle at my last assessment, I was still carrying 319 lb. on my joints, heart, lungs, etc.
- I was on blood thinners for the clot. The clot was later determined to be genetic, meaning that even if I got leaner and healthier, I'd take blood thinners the rest of my life.
- I was prediabetic and on my way to having full blown diabetes.
- I was out of "shape," just strong.
- My dad had heart disease and failure at age fifty-eight. He suffered for five years and passed at sixty-three. That wasn't far off for me.

I needed a new "why." I assessed and assessed. I talked with others, thought, and decided:

- I wanted to be able to walk my daughter down the aisle at her wedding. I wanted to see all my kids on their big days. I wanted to see them graduate.
- I wanted to feel better about my physical appearance.

- I wanted to be more active and hike the National Parks around the country. I specifically wanted to hike the Mohawk Lakes in Summit County, Colorado with Jen.
- I wanted to be in control of my life.
- Here is another big one: I was put on this Earth to help others learn to fight against their mental barriers and achieve their best levels of greatness. I believe this at my core as my calling. And this is why I opened my gym in 2013.
- I wanted to show people that I could play and win at racquetball for Purdue and weigh 190 lb., compete in strongman at age forty-five at 319 lb., and lose the weight and get back to a lean, strong version of myself before fifty.

These were my "whys." It was the next iteration of Jim Beebe. This was in the fourth quarter of 2021. It's now May of 2022 as I sit here writing in my basement. I weigh 270 lb. I'm on my way.

Here's the point for you. Write down your "whys" now. Take a few days and refine them. Talk with others. But dig deep into You. Make it real. Make it powerful. Then there are four more steps:

1. Keep them visible in at least six physical places.
2. Reevaluate monthly, quarterly, and annually. Go into your calendar now and schedule the days and times when you will do your assessments.
3. Share them with at least five people that are your allies. Not friends, but allies.
4. Things will happen in your life and your "Why" will change. Change with it. Change = Opportunity. Write that down too. Change = Opportunity.

The last piece is accountability. Always is. If I do this, then what? If I don't do this, then what? We will address the carrot and the stick metaphor later. All you need to know at this point is that pressure is a gift. And you must add it consistently and systematically to you. Always and often.

We improve what we measure. So first write down your "Whys". Then share them with your allies (step 3 above). The ally's task is asking you about your performance. He will want to know if you are executing. His knowing your "Why" alone adds a small bit of pressure that helps you move forward. Then tell the important people in your family. Again, more pressure. How you do anything is how you do everything. (You'll see that often in this book.) Then you'll start to live it out in your daily life. Your identity will evolve and become clearer. Your actions will follow your beliefs. It's why I'm authoring this book. I can help you get better! Follow me. Let's lock arms. Let's attack and move forward. Do this!

CHAPTER 2

BUILDING YOUR
MACHINE

Advancement and success require confidence. The adage "you have to believe to achieve" is true. Or "believe in yourself even if no one else does." Yup, also true. Still others instruct you to have confidence in yourself even before you've tried or done it, whatever "it" may be. Does that work? Well, yes and no.

For the most part, the answer is no. For most of you, the answer is no. It's a lie. Believe you can be an All-American when you're still a walk-on? C'mon. Really?! Unlikely, if not impossible. (When I use language like "impossible," I'm daring you to prove me wrong! I'd love nothing more than for you to contact me and say, "See! I did it!)

Ridiculous example: Are you confident you can drive your car entirely backward throughout the day? Not really. Possible? Yes. Probable? No. How about this: drive through your neighborhood completely backward for an hour. Then are you more confident in your ability to drive through your neighborhood backward? Yes, quite a bit more. Confidence only comes from reps! Bruce Lee said, "I don't fear that man that's practiced ten thousand different kicks. I fear the man that has practiced one singular kick ten thousand times." Reps, reps, reps.

Back to being a walk-on in college. Let's say it's for college soccer. How can you build your machine? How can you build your confidence? How can you build your brand and identity as a player that can play as an All-American? It's the same way anything is built. Copy it!

(At first.) Success leaves clues. And the clues aren't subtle either. The clues are screaming at you, like they are screaming in my head as I write this.

Then evolve what you copied. Make it better. Someone learned algebra. Then someone else evolved it and advanced it. Then someone evolved it and advanced to make geometry, trigonometry, calculus and so on. You must do the same thing to achieve your highest potential. Take all your lessons learned, all the ones I will teach you, everything you can think of in your sport, and advance that knowledge. You can do it. And if not you, then who? Because someone will.

Here is why you can't or won't become an All-American. Read this out loud to yourself. Or better yet, go to Wal-Mart, buy a megaphone, and scream it through the megaphone as you look at yourself in the mirror.

It takes massive, life-changing, family lineage-changing, generational wealth-changing work!

It will always come down to "Will you do the work?" If so, then you can. Otherwise. . . nope. No shortcuts. None. Go all in, and you can make it to the highest level. Follow the steps in this book, and you can. But you must work your ass off.

Context:

- Massive. What's massive? An elephant is massive. You may be putting in work that is the size of a nice golden retriever currently. You need an elephant-sized amount of work. And if one elephant is required, then you'd better make it two elephants.
- Family-lineage changing: That's the name on your back. Let's see if I say a name and you recognize it: Eisenstein, Jordan, Kobe, Washington, Caesar, Brady, Jesus (top of the list), Hitler. Anyone

going to know your last name? It takes the amount of work that makes people from all walks of life know your name.

• Generational wealth. Being an All-American means you're going pro. That means you're making millions. If you make $150,000 a year, you're in the top 5 percent in the world. What does millions per year equate to? Well, it's enough to affect you and your entire next generation of offspring. That level of wealth outlasts you (unless you're undisciplined with money) and your next generation. It takes that level of effort.

If you're still reading, then here's the deal: I'll spend the rest of this book and most of my life helping and showing anyone who'll listen to different processes and techniques for advancement. And with each small, incremental step—each "Inch"—you'll get better. Each time you improve, confidence builds. As confidence improves, you'll at least be confident enough to attempt harder and more monumental tasks. Accomplish one of those harder tasks, and confidence soars. Take on another fear or task or obstacle, yup, you guessed it. Boom, another win, and confidence grows. It's circular. It's beautiful and exciting when it's going in the right direction. It's terrifying and gut-wrenching going in the wrong direction. There is a process to keep moving forward. There is also a process for moving backward and regressing. You are the sum of your habits. Once you stop the positive momentum forward, there will be a time of pause. You'll plateau as your momentum ends. Then your momentum will pick up again. Only this time, it's back down the mountain you climbed. Your habits will take you to lower levels if you allow it to happen. So buckle in and hold on tight. And as if your life depended on it, keep moving forward! Get another Inch.

CHAPTER 3

IDENTITY

Who are you? It can take a lifetime to answer that question. It's also one thing to know yourself and completely another thing to let others know who you are. Authenticity, being real, wins. Fake loses. Both statements can be untrue in the short run, but it's an absolute truth in the long run. So, I'll ask again, who are you? What are you about? Then where do you want to go?

Painful example. I was finishing up my junior year at St. Ignatius High School in Cleveland. I did well in math and science, and I had to struggle tooth and nail for grades in other subjects. There were plenty of reminders, too, for successes and failures. I had my GPA, my class ranking, and the question of which colleges could be a good fit for me. I also had the "gift" of the $50 penalty from my parents each semester. This meant that for every grade I received below an A-, I had to pay $50 toward my tuition. So, a B+ was $50, a B was $100, etc. This was for each class. This sucked and was total bullshit. And sometimes circumstances are total bullshit. And it does not matter. You must still move forward. What else will you do—quit? I can't. I won't. But it's also true with life. Execution is rewarded. Failure is not. The end.

Here's the real painful part: I knew that after college I wanted to go into some sort of business, investments, or even run my own business. I just didn't know what that form would take. That's okay. That's what college is for. The problem was that my science teachers, advisors, and some family members strongly suggested I study engineering because of my abilities in math and science. It was logical. As a result, I went against myself and my gut and ultimately enrolled Purdue University for engineering. This was no one else's fault. I decided. It was my choice.

I started college in the fall of 1993, and it was an out-of-state school. That was $17,000/year at the time. My father said he'd pay for my college education. Near the end of my second semester, he was out of money, so I had to earn money on my own, which I did. Now I was entering my third semester, paying my way to start my sophomore year in a major I didn't want! And after three semesters total at Purdue, I was "invited not to return to engineering." I quickly transferred to the business school. That was where I should have been from the start. I had lied to myself. And lies always come out. Pain. Inexcusable pain. Completely avoidable pain if only I had been honest with myself, who I was, and where I wanted to go.

You must do the same thing. Be honest with yourself fully. And then be honest with others fully. It's the only way that's sustainable. Listen to yourself. Use your brain and your heart. Never rely solely on one. That's always a losing approach. Take a breath. Write out the issue. Figure it out. And be real! Be who you are and go forward. It's your only shot.

As you progress through this book, keep this question in mind: Who are you? You are dynamic, not static. That means that over time you will change and evolve. Who you were as a young child will be different from who you are as a parent of two kids in the middle of a career. You will learn things about yourself as you read and apply the principles in this book. Take note of that. Embrace who you are. But stay true to your Core Values, and go with it. Hard. With passion and resolve. Move forward.

What values do you have? I listed the six you must have (Integrity, Discipline, Kaizen, Teamwork, Enjoyment, Sisu), plus the overall mantra to apply them (Relentlessness). Do you agree? You won't go wrong if you apply those values Relentlessly. But ask yourself is there another one that matters to you? If so, great! Ask yourself why. Then know it, believe it, act on it.

I don't mind so much what your habits or actions have been in the past. Take another moment and assess what your strengths and weaknesses are in terms of the six Core Values and/or your own Core Values. How do you stack up consistently? Then where must we go next in applying your Core Values?

For example, Discipline is a Core Value. We can agree that being early to every practice is critical for an athlete. If you don't do that, you lack Discipline in this instance. And that habit must improve for you to remain true to your identity. It also must occur if you hope to play at all. That's an easy example. Take it a step further. In football, you're running with the threes (you're third string) on defense, and you have been jumping offsides. Undisciplined. You won't climb the depth chart and could get knocked down if this continues. Do you stay after practice for thirty minutes working on snap drills to improve? That take Discipline. Do you continue this for two weeks, so that it never occurs again? Discipline. The loser only practices until he gets it right. The winner practices enough that he never gets it wrong. 100 percent unwavering Discipline.

I am not suggesting you must always have Discipline in every aspect of your life. That's not sustainable. We make errors, slack off, and relent at times. But I will insist that you strive to apply Discipline for you to get to where you want to be. You will fail. Fine. But keep striving to apply that value. In fact, overapply that value and see where you end up. Discipline alone will take you extremely far. The same is exactly true for all your Core Values and the six I listed previously. Relentlessly strive to apply your Core Values in the future. This will keep you grounded and in check.

Future: Your Future Self
-Where do you want to be in twelve months?
-Stop right there. Words are not everything, but they are important.

Do this instead:

-Where would you like to be in twelve months? Nope, that's crap.

-Where do you want to be in twelve months? Better version of crap.

-Where must you be in twelve months? Tony Robbins version.

This is awesome.

Here's my version: Where must you be? Where is it that I'd be stupid not to be in 12 months? Where is it that if I'm not there in twelve months, I'd be so disgusted with myself and disappointed that I'd do anything to get there?

This is not "I want to be all-conference in high school football or college football." Those are your targets and milestones on your journey. We will shoot for those and get there, but this question is bigger than those milestones. I am on a much bigger path. You are on a much bigger path. You are climbing this mountain that only culminates on your deathbed. And then your legacy takes over from there. Between now and then is the next year. What kind of person, athlete, entity must you become in the twelve months that leads you to where you want to be at the top of your mountain?

Read that paragraph again.

Where must you be in the next twelve months that nothing will stop you from achieving your goals?

Then, what milestones must you pass in the next twelve months? Future projects? Stop. Think. Write it down.

What will that mean to you? You will evolve and grow. You will accomplish tasks and hit targets. What will that mean to you? Write that down.

What does that feel like? Confidence up? You betcha! Beliefs improve? Of course. Might you simply feel happy? Duh. Let's say you start at third on the depth chart (third string) and move to the second string. Then the starter goes down due to injury. Your number gets called. The second half of the season goes by, and you're clearly the starter going forward. It happens all the time. It's the Wally Pip scenario. Wally Pip gets hurt playing first base for the New York Yankees. Lou Gherig gets his number called to step up. Now Gherig is a "Statue" guy and never relinquished his spot until he retired. He played in 2,130 straight games in fifteen years, never missing a game. He's a Hall of Famer with his name, statue, and legacy in many places. Write down how you'd feel then.

Next, make two lists. What obstacles are in the way? What tools do you need to get there? Ask your coaches; ask your teammates. Get clarity on what is necessary. It's okay if you're not aware. . . for now. For now, approach it like this. What obstacles and tools do you have in the following areas:

- Mindset
- Knowledge
- Teammates
- Training
- Nutrition
- Recovery

In the future chapters, we will explore and identify your needs. We will know one way or another what you must do to improve. Guaranteed. For now, think broadly about where you must be in twelve months.

CHAPTER 4

CORE VALUES INTRODUCTION

As far as Core Values go, get your own. ☺ These are mine. Mine are tried and true. They work well for me. My gym uses our Core Values to guide how we operate and govern our business. But here's the thing: Each one must speak to you. Each must align with your identity. When one is out of line with your actions, you feel it. Core Values are the words that stand for the actions you take when people are watching and when no one is. Adversity doesn't test your character; it reveals it. You can copy and implement the Core Values presented here, or you can pick completely different ones. However, you must choose three to six and adhere to them. Your Core Values will keep you centered and guide you when making decisions and acting on them.

Task

Take five minutes. Calm yourself and shut your eyes. Think about who you are. Think about what your family stands for, good and bad. Think about what your team stands for, good and bad. Think about what you must be known for doing. Think about how you must be known for living. Think about your personality now and your future personality. Who are you now? And who will you evolve to over time? What components or characteristics are important? Write them down.

After that task, try to combine any candidates that are duplicative. Look for overlap. For example, Discipline, Diligence, and Perseverance are synonyms. So, pick only one. Narrow the field next and shrink the list down to your top ten.

Next, pick one Core Value. In this example, let's select Loyalty as a potential candidate. Then take those thoughts through this iteration.

1. I can be loyal.
2. I should be known for being loyal.
3. I will be known for being loyal.
4. I must be known for being loyal.
5. I'd be crazy and stupid if I weren't known for being loyal.
6. I am loyal. I am a loyal person, a loyal teammate, a loyal worker, and a loyal family member or friend.

If you make it to the sixth statement and believe it, then there is a good chance this could be one of your Core Values. Now wash, rinse, repeat. Run all your Core Value candidates through this iteration and see which rise to the top and which fade away. Once you have your list, the rest of your life will be the lab in which you stress test each Core Value. For example, you decided that Loyalty is one of yours, and your teammate constantly asks you to show up for early morning workouts with him. The first time you miss could be a simple accident or oversight. The second and third times might mean you're lazy, have a weak "Why," or simply don't care. But each time you say you'll be there for your friend and teammate, and don't. . . Well, you're clearly not loyal in this instance. Either Loyalty is a Core Value, or it hasn't been one for you lately. In which case you must re engage and lock that one in permanently. Check yourself and get back to living your life how you believed you'd be "crazy and stupid if you weren't a loyal teammate." Either you are loyal, or you are not. Perfection is impossible, but if Loyalty is You, then live it and do it.

You'll notice that several words are always capitalized in this book. It's the important ones. What are the Core Values of *Athlete Builder*? What are my Core Values? They are one and the same. Professionally, they are as follows. To become the athlete you want to be, you'll need at least the same professional Core Values listed here. Add any more that you need as well.

Integrity
Discipline
Kaizen
Teamwork
Enjoyment
Sisu

Furthermore, to my personal Core Values, I add the following:

Faith
Family
Health

The overarching mantra that I apply to each Core Value is

Relentless

Each value must be applied Relentlessly. It's not a "sometime thing." You can't become a "little bit pregnant." You either are or you aren't. Now, am I perfect at achieving and holding true to my Core Values every day? Nope. But it is the directive, nonetheless. And when I struggle with decisions, these values point me in the right direction. But you must be Relentless if you are to get anywhere. Here is one of my favorite examples. My daughter, Maddie, earned five years of a full-ride academic scholarship to the University of Alabama. One of her many AP classes her junior year in high school was AP Chemistry. She's prepared for all her exams Relentlessly and earned a 5 (highest score possible) on the Chem exam. I asked her what her process was. She said she reviewed all her year's notes and prior exams, of course. And her teacher gave her the last twenty years of prior AP exams. I casually asked if she did a few of them or a few questions in certain sections over the twenty prior exams. She laughed at me and my approach. "Of course not, Dad. I did them all. I did all twenty exams. Then I knew that when I took the final test, I was fully prepared." Confidence only comes from reps. She did all the reps and earned her confidence and her results. Relentless.

CHAPTER 5

INTEGRITY

The All Blacks are New Zealand's rugby team and the most successful franchise in Earth's history. They have a higher lifetime winning percentage of matches than any team in any sport, over 75 percent. This is for over a hundred years! One of their many mantras is, "Sweep the sheds." James Kerr highlights it in his book, *Legacy*. After a basic practice, when the players are exhausted and beat up, they each start with the chores of leaving their place in better shape than they found it. They "sweep the sheds" to clean up everything. When they finish competing in a test (the rugby term for a game or match), they "sweep the sheds" of their locker room at home and away games. It's fundamental to their culture of doing their best in all things regardless of how they feel. How you do anything is how you do everything.

Integrity: It comes from the word *integer*. It's singular or whole with you. It "feels right" with you. It's doing what is right, always. For me, it's "How you do anything is how you do everything." It's a lifestyle. It's for all components of your life: health, relationships, faith, moral code, work ethic, and your effort. It's not perfection. It's striving to do your best in all endeavors.

This Core Value leads things off because it leads all other Core Values. It leads to what we do and what we are to become. Taking on this Core Value is so powerful that it will guide you where you want to be without knowing much else. Simply do your best at everything. I can make a case that you don't need to know anything more than that if you apply that value Relentlessly. Act with Integrity in your Training, your Nutrition, your Recovery, your Mindset, your Knowledge of your sport, and your relationships with your Teammates, and you're virtually set. Put this book down and get to work. Integrity alone will guide you a very long way.

Let's be specific here. Let's quantify and clarify what Integrity "looks like" and is for an athlete. This list is not comprehensive or exhaustive. It's the basics.

- Are you on time to practice, meetings, games, class, etc.? On time is good. It's the minimum. I'm fifteen minutes early. Which are you? Which is your standard?
- Do you stop when you're tired or when you're done? Did you run that sprint through the line or stop short? Getting to the line is good. Going beyond is better. Going all out and beyond the line is best. Doing that every time is doing your best and acting with Integrity. What's your standard?
- You're exhausted from college two-a-days, and you're cleaning up to head home. How's your locker room? Did you leave your towels on the floor and your locker in disarray? Or are you squared away? Did you pick up anyone else's towels, so the place is as good as you found it or better? Did you remind your teammates to get squared away as well? Which are you? You have Integrity or you don't. Your team has Integrity in this instance, or it doesn't. You're part of that team. If the team doesn't, then you don't. Raise your standard of Integrity.
- It's the week of your championship game. You're in a new city and the team is playing on national TV. You're the starting point guard for your basketball team. Are you out getting drunk one night that week leading up to the game? Or are you preparing for the game? Are you getting your teammates to bed on time? Are you making sure you're fed, hydrated, and rested properly? Are

you spending time watching more film so you're overprepared? What's your standard? Raise your level of Integrity.

Let's be clear. You're not reading this book so you can be good. Good is a fine aspiration for the average person. It's not for me, and it's not for this book. Good is getting by. I don't want to be great either. I want you to be legendary. What does that mean? For example, if that means the absolute best you can do on a math exam is 93 percent given your abilities and work ethic, then I want 93.1 percent. I want whatever you can do at your purest form and effort, plus a little more. That's legendary. It's standing up from that back squat with your body shaking, almost shitting yourself, with your eyes about to pop out with five more pounds on the bar than you ever even imagined you could do. And it's not one of those bitch-squats either that is only a quarter of the way down. It must be legit. I can already figure out what you can do. I want you to go beyond that, to that point you only dreamed of going.

That level of achievement is true greatness. That doesn't mean you made the team, or you were a starter, an all-pro, or even in the Hall of Fame. That level is only particular to you and you surpassing your abilities. None of that occurs without Integrity and doing your best. And write this down: Whatever you're doing now is not your best. You can do more. So do it. Thousands of years and generations have occurred on this planet to give you the last name on your back. Don't embarrass yourself and your family legacy by not fulfilling your destiny. Live with Integrity. Go out there and Relentlessly crush the next task in front of you.

CHAPTER 6

DISCIPLINE = FREEDOM

Wish I had produced this equation myself. I wasn't smart enough or clever enough to word it. But Jocko Willink is the author of the phrase. And he is spot on. It's painted on a wall at Unbreakable Athletics. I say it often. I study and learn and go through other masters' notes and "rules" or "laws". Then I apply them Relentlessly for growth and improvement. Jocko's equation is sound, and it is true. Adopt it for yourself and advance. Don't, and you will peril your chance. Choose. And choose today.

Think about it. Even better, meditate on it. Here is the timeless formula from your geometry class. Most don't love math, but I do. My mother was a great high school math teacher, and I've always loved it. So bear with me. It'll make sense, I promise.

If P, then Q.

For this equation, if certain things are true, then the result must be true. Simple example in math: If a four-sided object has all four sides of equal length and each angle is 90 degrees, then the object is a square. Simple equation in sports: If the Cleveland Browns score 21 points in a game and the Pittsburgh Steelers score 20, then the Browns won. Of course, in reality this is a rare occasion. But it's still true.

For Jocko, you, me, and the world, if you have Discipline, then you will have Freedom.

Real life example for Maddie Beebe. If her PSAT and SAT scores are high enough to make her a National Merit Finalist, then she will have the freedom to attend the University of Alabama for five years with every expense paid and an added $3,500/year stipend. True story. Academic Discipline = academic and financial freedom. In 2022, she hit all her test score requirements and received her full scholarship. Earned. Not given.

Another example: You are obese with high blood sugar; you will either be prediabetic or diabetic. If you are Disciplined with your health, diet, and training, then you can have the freedom to be off medications and healthy. If you do P, then you will receive Q.

The issue is that for total freedom, it usually takes Discipline in more than one area. But the equation still holds. The trick is finding all the factors that make up the P side of the equation to satisfy the Q side. What does that look like? Examples:

- If you're enrolled in college with the required GPA, and
- If you're the best size for middle linebacker, and
- If you're the strongest, fastest, and most explosive middle linebacker, and
- If you know the playbook the best, and
- If you have the best Nutrition and Recovery system, and
- If you have the strongest work ethic, and
- If you have the best attitude and are the most supportive Teammate, and
- If you own the toughest and most focused Mindset, and
- If you can make plays better than anyone else at middle linebacker,
- THEN, you get the freedom to start at middle linebacker for your team. Likewise,

- If you're the best in the conference, then you get the freedom of being All-Conference.
- If you're the best in the nation, then you get the freedom of being an All-American.
- If you're an All-American, then you'll get the freedom from being drafted.
- If you're the best in the NFL, then you'll get the freedom of being All-Pro.
- If you're a ten-time All-Pro, then you'll get the freedom of being a Hall of Famer. You will be at the Statue level for an athlete.

And this is only in your line of work, your field of endeavor. Apply this to your faith. Apply this to your relationship with your spouse, and to parenthood if you're eventually a mother or father. Apply this Relentlessly and watch your freedoms unfold.

Tangibly, what does this mean? What does this look like as an athlete? Score yourself in the first eight bullet points listed above. Then find your weaknesses is each area. Prioritize your biggest weakness in each area. Then schedule time each day to work solely on your eight biggest weaknesses. Reevaluate each week, month, quarter, and year. Adjust and execute, Relentlessly. Share this with an accountability ally. Over-execute! "Moderation is for cowards." – US Navy SEALs.

There is a systematic process for this. And you have it in your hands. I will lay it out for you. And you will advance. This is going to be great. Just keep moving forward through this book. Take as many notes as possible. We'll get there, I promise.

CHAPTER 7

KAIZEN

What in the what? What does this mean? Why here? Have you ever seen athletes or generals or whoever author a book? They draw parallels from the lessons learned on the field of battle or the court and field of play. They apply those parallels to life lessons and to personal and professional endeavors. Why? How can that be? Well, you saw in the section on Discipline, that there are equations or rules and laws that apply universally. The same is true here.

In 2008, I went back to Purdue for my master's degree. I received a master of science in finance in twelve months. Most MBA programs take twenty-four months to complete. Kaizen is Japanese, and it's also a business term I learned at Purdue University. Summed up, it means to look for improvement in all matters relevant to your endeavor. It's the "1 percent at a time" mantra you read about. Why? The compound interest effect is our process for creating greatness. When we identify the priority for each of the six components, we have a shot at improvement. Then we must work tirelessly to evolve and progress at least 1 percent more in each priority. Doing so advances you as an athlete, person, or team. The ultimate goal is to win, and adopting this core value guides us to facilitate winning.

How do I sum this concept up? The answer:

HUNT WEAKNESSES.

Read Ray Dalio's book, *Principles*. The entire premise is that he, his company, his culture—everything in his life—is set up to hunt for weaknesses in all processes. It's the feedback loop, and it is necessary for success. Here are ways to apply it: First and foremost, take a critical look at your processes as an athlete, student, employee, family member. Find the priority weakness in each endeavor. Make a small adjustment to each process to improve it. Keep doing it until it's an ingrained habit. Then run the process again. Do this forever until you die. Simple, not easy.

Here's another way to apply it when there isn't a problem per se. Often, I'll unfortunately see coaches agonizing over the program they're writing for the athletes. So much time and anxiety occur in the process. This is where the US Navy SEAL mantra, "A good plan today is better than a perfect plan tomorrow," needs to kick in. That means spending time and producing as good a plan or program for training as you can design in one day. Then immediately implement it and get feedback from athletes by seeing the results. Then adjust on the fly for that session and alter it for future sessions. I can take a good plan and get ten iterations of it in under two weeks. Others haven't even tried their "perfect plan" over the two-week period. Meanwhile I'm so far down the road, I can't even see that person behind me.

As an athlete, you must hunt your weaknesses to evolve. Taking a Relentless approach with this simple—not easy—Core Value will propel you further than you can picture right now. There is always a progression and next step. Move forward and find it.

Spoiler alert: The last section of this book is the method for constant improvement. Kaizen. If you can't figure out a process to do everything mentioned above, don't worry at all. I have it taken care of for you. You must simply supply Relentless effort.

CHAPTER 8

TEAMWORK

There is a phrase on our gym wall: "Strength of the pack is the wolf. And the strength of the wolf is the pack." There are a multitude of phrases or quotes to illustrate this point. The wolf pack theme is one of our favorites. It's also said that if you want to go fast, then go alone. But if you want to go far, then go together. Or, if you want to see your future, then show me the five people you spend time with the most. Are you starting to get a feel of where we are going with this Core Value? No one, and I mean no one, does it alone. Pick any of the greats and look them up. Each had a coach. Each had a Teammate to push them. Each had to learn from someone. No one comes out of the womb great. If you can accomplish your goals alone, then you have very small goals. Larger goals require a Team.

Example in nature: the wolf pack. They hunt, travel, and live as a group. There's a leader, the alpha. There are the stronger and weaker, older and younger of wolves within the group. Google "wolf pack traveling ranks." You'll see a multitude of people sharing the same picture and post via Facebook, Instagram, etc. There are twenty-four wolves traveling in a single-file line through the snow. The first three are the oldest and sickest. They set the pace. If they didn't set the pace and the healthier, stronger groups did, then the old and sick are left behind. Next in line are the five strongest on alert. The strongest are looking for threats and opportunities. The next five strongest are at the back doing the same thing from a different vantage point. All other "troops" save one are between the ten strongest marching along in formation. The lone alpha male is at the rear, assessing all components of the team. He's there for any rear ambush. He watches over the pack and understands the pace within the environment. The entire group is one unit. It's life and death.

Example in sports (Honestly, do we even really need to go through this exercise? No one wins alone!): Take the greatest of the greatest. Pick anyone. It won't matter.

Michael Jordan. He had HOF coach Dean Smith at University of North Carolina, HOF coach Bobby Knight on the USA Olympic team, HOF coach Phil Jackson with the Chicago Bulls, HOF trainer Tim Grover, HOF players Scottie Pippen and Dennis Rodman, a support crew for his personal affairs. Heck, he had someone in charge of his garage. The garage attendant detailed his car perfectly each day.

How about an individual sport like golf? Tiger Woods. His father, Earl, molded his golf skills from an early age and brought his Mindset skills along even further than his physical skills. Tiger always had a coach and a caddy to help him. He has a team for his branding, investments, deals, etc. The list goes on and on.

Here's a tough one. How about Bobby Fisher, the US chess prodigy and all-time great? It's truly a loner sport. And when you are on the top of the mountain, it's singular and lonely. Your only help comes from those who are at that level mentally. So yes, he had help early on in his life. At an early age, someone taught him and coached him in his sport. Later in life, his only real help came from other historical chess legends, and this was only through their writings and books. So, did he really have help from a team? Yes. He did. He realized that the mental strain associated with competing in this sport affected him physically. The opposite was also true. Physical preparedness improved his mental preparedness. So, he got a coach who had him swimming and exercising so he was in top shape to compete mentally. Inches. Everything matters.

As a Teammate, you have important duties. Your job and role are to get "squared away" first and lead by example. Next, influence those in your inner circle. If you're the center back in soccer, then get the entire back row to meetings early like you do. Impart your knowledge to them. Get them better! Once this is complete, expand and permeate to the next part of the team until all are on board. Keep applying this Relentlessly.

Hold yourself accountable and to the highest standards. Then hold Teammates to their highest standards as well as to the team standards. Don't ask, "How are things going?" It's too easy and too broad. Ask, "What's not going well with your Training? What's not going well with your Recovery?" Listen. Understand it. "Get it." Then either solve the issue or find a solution from another resource.

You must also recognize that you are a Teammate with your leadership. That means coaches, assistant coaches, teachers, professors, bosses, etc. Are you coachable or not? This relationship is everything. Otherwise, you won't improve enough to win. And that's the point of playing, to win. Work hard at listening and applying what you're asked to do. Work to understand and clarify. It's a process, and you must work at it.

At the same time, do not take for granted your support staff. The assistants, cleaning crew, family and friends, agents, etc. all work for your benefit in some capacity. In all relationships, a simple "please" and "thank you" go a very long way. And find a way to give something back. Being a Teammate is a two-way street that's always moving. You must keep at it, so your relationships are strong and worthwhile.

The goal is to make your Teammates better, and I mean better than even you. This includes all Teammates at all levels. Why? Well, you're competitive. (If not, put the book down. This isn't for you.) But with better Teammates, you must elevate yourself to catch and surpass them again. And just like that, everyone evolves to their next iteration. It's beautiful.

CHAPTER 9

ENJOYMENT

James Clear highlights in his book, *Atomic Habits*, that certain things must occur for new habits to start and persist. (Make habits easy, attractive, easy, and satisfying.) And one necessity is Enjoyment. Combining Clear's approach to building habits with our prior Core Values will make new habits more enjoyable for you. We are "selling" restraint, work, struggle, and effort at Unbreakable Athletics. The same is true with this book *Athlete Builder*. We are not selling beer, pizza, and entertainment. We ask everyone to work here, to work hard! Almost no one would stick with us if there weren't a level of Enjoyment with our approach. It's hot here in the summer—over 100 degrees Fahrenheit. And no one likes to leave their house in the winter. And those obstacles get trumped when athletes have a strong "Why" for being here. It helps to make it fun as well. And honestly, the best way to have a fun time with a grueling task is to have a funny, engaging personality with your Teammates. That will help the most.

We crank the music up. We have contests. We host events and competitions. We raise money for charities. We laugh at our mistakes. We ring the PR (personal record) bell when we succeed. We wear ridiculous outfits. We cheer each other on when the struggle gets real. The team looks for the struggle. We learn to enjoy discomfort because we know it's the only path to growth. "Oh man, this is going to suck, let's get it." Who says that? I've seen ladies in here with their pants on backward and inside out. And guys the same goes for their shorts. And sometimes no one bothers to change because it's funny and no one cares. Entire classes go to parties or go shopping together. I've seen an entire class go on a week-long vacation together. This would only happen if we enjoyed what we are doing and with whom we are doing it. That's the culture at Unbreakable. Enjoyment and Teamwork go hand in hand.

"Be thankful for the struggle, for it creates perseverance." – 1 James.

Early in June of 2022 (one week ago as I'm writing this), an athlete was in my office in tears. His fiancé and soon-to-be mother of his daughter broke off the relationship. In addition, he suffered an injury competing at rugby that ended his career. Two major plans he had had for himself were set back, damaging him and his identity.

Similarly, a coach was in my office and had "lost her way" and identity with her training, her personal endeavors, and her financial endeavors because of the deteriorating economy in 2022.

What does this have to do with Enjoyment? Neither situation is fun or even close to optimal. I sat there and listened and identified with them. I easily remembered my own struggles. As a quick example, I went to Purdue University for my undergraduate degree. I was from Ohio, so the cost was "out of state" and a big deal for me and my family. My parents were divorced. My mother's side said they would not help with any costs. My dad said he'd cover it alone. Halfway through my second semester, Dad said he had no more money. If I had known that, I would've gone to a cheaper school in the state. Now I was at a crossroads. What would I do? Drop out and work, stay at Purdue, transfer to an Ohio school, or what? God chose for me. I received a letter in the mail, a solicitation. Would you, Jim Beebe, like to run a painting franchise for College Pro Painters? You'll learn how to run a business and earn money along the way. I was at a low. But I'm also a risk-taker. So, I said "yes." Long story short, I grossed over $60,000 in revenue in the summer of 1995 and had enough to pay for my schooling. It's a period that I am proud of and look back on fondly because of my struggles and perseverance. The pain and discomfort facilitated growth for me. I had to adapt and overcome. I become stronger and more resilient. I had a fun time with my crew and friends while doing it. I ended up enjoying the process and benefited greatly from it.

Here's the point. Be thankful for the struggle, for it creates perseverance. Enjoy it. Nowadays I must fabricate struggles and challenges to grow. I must make them up! If I were in a dark place, a vicious hole, then I'd be in the middle of evolving, of getting stronger, or improving. I love that. But growth only comes from the struggle.

My two friends and athletes above are in the middle of their struggles. And it was a struggle that would make everyone better if managed well. In a sick, perverse way, I was jealous. I was happy for them because this instance and opportunity was their chance to improve. As in the movie *Gladiator*, "When death smiles at you, all you can do is smile back." So, find some happiness in the struggle. Seek discomfort. How did they turn out? Well, the rugby player moved on and is now a rugby coach for a high school team doing very well. It was time for him to move on to a different role. My other coach also moved on to her original gym back in her hometown. Both found different options that were still challenging but also enjoyable as well. It's a requirement for sustainability.

In David Goggins *Can't Hurt Me*, he discusses the concept of taking souls. It internally puts a smile on his face, and it will do the same for you. This only occurs during and within the struggle. Find joy in it.

Ask Jack Beebe about the summer of 2022. At the end of conditioning sessions for Ball State football, he was beating his teammates handily in the conditioning drills. He later said he was smiling just looking around at everyone while he was performing and suffering in the heat. Finding a piece of joy in the struggle made it easier for him to compete and enabled him to elevate his performance. Then doing it again the next day became easier and more fun. A new habit was forming, and a lesson was learned.

Find joy in what you do. It matters.

CHAPTER 10

SISU

This word was my first tattoo. Ink Therapy in Plainfield, Indiana hooked me up. The word is a mantra and cultural staple for the country of Finland. The Beebe name is not Finnish but Scottish and English. So why *Sisu*? You'll need to look this one up, too. There isn't a literal English translation. For me, it's summed up as this: When you're really at the end of your rope, ready to commit suicide, despondent, hopeless, and ready quit, then Sisu means keep going and never quit. Ever.

Don't ever quit. Ever. There's no respect in it. Don't quit on yourself, your Teammates, or your family. The end. We could leave it at that and be "good" if we always applied this Core Value Relentlessly. However, there is a little bit more. There is always a little bit more.

When you're at your worst, it's obvious and natural to say, "Don't quit." It not easy; it's brutally hard. But it's also simple. Take one step forward. Don't think; just do. Move forward. That's it. But also look at this scenario: The task is max rep back squats at 225 lb., leaving one or two reps in the tank. All right. For the 275 lb. max squatter, this probably means four to six reps at this weight. Well, what if you're a 500 lb. squatter? That number of reps should surpass thirty! Whoa?! That is painful. That is hard cardio. That's an easy one to say "I did fifteen or twenty reps. That was hard. I'm good." But that's wrong. You know you had at least ten more in you. And you punked out. That kind of "quitting" isn't as obvious but is at least as damaging. All in, or not at all!

If the drill is to run to the line, then run to it or beyond it. Don't quit early. Sisu means never quit. Ever! If you tell your teammate you're coming over tonight, then don't "ghost him" and not show up. Don't quit on him. Be there. Integrity is coming into play here as well, another Core Value.

At its most basic level, Sisu keeps you off the bottom rung of your life and keeps you surviving. Sometimes this is all you can do. That's okay; stay on your path and continue forward. But you're looking for more than that. The thriving level of grit gets developed next. That level requires you to stay with the required task longer, more deliberately, and more fully than others. It means that you're the first to get to your training and the last to leave, getting everything addressed. It means getting your food prepped and film watched. It means maximizing your sleep and helping your teammates with their tasks too. The challenge is not quitting on the task but "winning" every task every day. This application of Sisu takes the athlete from surviving to thriving and is the separator of greatness for everyone.

It's why everyone loves Rocky. He didn't quit and always went to the final bell. Always. Even the motto of the Goonies is "Never say die!" Here is a recent example: Look up Rich Strike in the 2022 Kentucky Derby. The video and call are outstanding. The horse was an eighty to one shot. There was a late scratch, and a new horse, Rich Strike, entered the last twenty-four hours to run in the race. The course is 1.25 miles, and after 1.0 miles Rich Strike was sitting in fifteenth place out of twenty horses. The jockey moved the horse to the rail and started to weave as it hit a massive kick to sprint to the end. The announcer was about to call the favorite the winner when in the last couple seconds, Rich Strike barely took the lead and won the race by half a horse length. Epic.

What's that like personally for me? Too many examples to count. None of mine were as impressive as Rich Strike. In March of 2013, I opened my gym. At the time it was CrossFit Unbreakable. Today it's evolved to Unbreakable Athletics Academy. Early on, my banker lied to me about my financing. I secured half the money needed to start up the business, kicked in five percent myself, and the bank was to supply the rest if I held up my end. He lied and lied, leading me on. Long story short, no money came from his bank. This made the rest of 2013 very hard because my business was underfunded. It left me in a dire situation.

In addition, usually in January the "New Year's resolution" crowd comes into the gym. Well, in January of 2014 the governor of Indiana closed the state because of the winter blizzard. Newbies didn't come in at all because they couldn't. Veteran gym members quit too because it was closed. So, now I was stacking up losses without the funding from the bank there to support me. My only funding from personal lenders was set at 14 percent interest rate + 3 percent of all revenue. It was a deal only someone desperate to make it would do. And I was desperate. Some days it came down to buying gas or food. And one late night, I had to pay cash to the repo guy on my doorstep who was about to tow my car away. This was tremendous pain for me and my three kids. I had joint custody at the time with my ex-wife. Fortunately, she was supportive and accommodating of my situation at the time. The overall situation was not sustainable. I must adapt and overcome.

Fast forward to present day, June 2022 as I write this section. Each year has been bigger and more profitable than the prior. We service more and more members each day and enjoy doing it. For several years, the only thing I could do was keep my head down and never quit. Know this: Only 4 percent of all new businesses make it ten years. I'm hitting that next March easily. Sisu mindset got me through it. It will do the same for you.

CHAPTER 11

INCHES ASSESSMENT TEST

There are three things to note about the Assessment Test. First, like a company's quarterly financials, the score is a snapshot in time. Meaning, it's your score on this day only. Second, tomorrow the score can change, quickly. Simply letting your Teammates know your "Why" tomorrow will take your score from 0 on up. Third, you can complete other tasks like finding an accountability ally for the Inch Blocks. That will raise your score as well. The point is that you can make improvements quickly. And you will. Don't worry one minute about it. I got you. I have the method for success.

Your scoring trend is more important over time than your score today. You must increase your averages each quarter. Quickly. Do this and see where you are. See where your confidence will be. Watch yourself win! We will Relentlessly execute your plan. Let your Kaizen habit lead the way.

Take the Inches Assessment quarterly. You can take it alone or collaborate with a teammate, ally, mentor, or coach. Be honest and accurate. Keep a record of your score each time. The Overall section looks at your results for the last season and/or the last three months. This section won't always change each quarter. Regardless, still complete it. For multiple questions, your answer may be between two different criteria (e.g., between six and four points). If that's the case, then select the average (five points).

Simply answer the questions the best you can. If you do not know something or understand a concept yet, don't worry about it. Simply keep reading along in the book, and you'll learn everything. Then retake the test. Retake it as often as you like and see where you can improve quickly. And keep at it.

ˌOVERALL

What percent of games did your team win?

Your score is the percent rounded down (e.g., If you won 69.999 percent of games, your score would be 6).

POINTS: _____

What "All" were you? Were you All-State, All-American, All-Conference, etc.?

- 10 Points: First Team All-American or All-State
- 9 Points: Second Team All-American or All-State
- 8 Points: Third Team All-American or All-State
- 7 Points: First Team All-Conference
- 6 Points: Second Team All-Conference
- 5 Points: Third Team All-Conference
- 4 Points: Captain
- 0 Points: Anything else

POINTS: _____

What is your position on the team's depth chart?

- 10 Points: First Team
- 8 Points: Second Team
- 6 Points: Third Team
- 4 Points: Fourth Team
- 0 Points: Anything else

POINTS: _____

TOTAL POINTS: _____

OVERALL AVERAGE (TOTAL POINTS / 3) _____

Next, we will assess your Mindset. This is a broad category and the most critical. Your Mindset compels you to move forward. If you have a solid Mindset, then you will do the necessary things to advance. Let's see how you do.

<u>MINDSET</u>

How well do you and others know your "Why"?

- 10 Points: You know it; your unit knows it; your team knows it; your coaches know it; your support team knows it. You review it daily.
- 8 Points: Two groups mentioned above know it. You review it at least four times a week.

- 6 Points: You and your immediate Teammates know it. You review it weekly.
- 4 Points: You know it and review it monthly.
- 2 Points: You know it and review it quarterly.

POINTS: _____

How well do you and others know your Core Values?

- 10 Points: You know it; your unit knows it; your team knows it; your coaches know it; your support team knows it. You review it weekly.
- 8 Points: Two groups mentioned above know it. You review it at least weekly.
- 6 Points: You and your immediate Teammates know it. You review it weekly.
- 4 Points: You know it and review it monthly.
- 2 Points: You know it and review it quarterly.

POINTS: _____

What is your level of Integrity?

- 10 Points: You give maximum effort (90 percent or more) daily.
- 8 Points: You give 80 percent effort daily.
- 3 Points: You give 60 percent effort daily.
- 0 Points: All else.

POINTS: _____

What is your level of Enjoyment? How well do you reflect on positives, have gratitude, act humble, help others, and ultimately enjoy your sport?

- 10 Points: Daily
- 8 Points. Weekly
- 6 Points. Monthly
- 4 Points. Quarterly
- 0 Points: All else.

POINTS: _____

Sisu

- 10 Points: You never quit, ever. You push through all reps, see tasks to completion and beyond.
- 8 Points: You mostly complete all tasks to the fullest.
- 5 Points: You occasionally complete tasks to the fullest.
- 0 Point: All else.

POINTS: _____

Discipline

- 10 Points: You consistently do what must be done, when it must be done, beyond the minimums.
- 8 Points: You mostly do what must be done when it must be done.
- 5 Points: You occasionally do what must be done when it must be done.
- 0 Points: All else.

POINTS: _____

Kaizen

- 10 Points: You have a process for improving and adhere to it without fail.
- 8 Points: You mostly have a process and adhere to it.
- 5 Points: You occasionally have a process and adhere to it.
- 0 Points: All else.

POINTS: _____

Mindset Mentor

- 10 Points: You have one and connect weekly.
- 8 Points: You have one and connect monthly.
- 5 Points: You have one and connect quarterly.
- 0 Points: All else.

POINTS: _____

How effectively are you working with a Mindset accountability ally (or allies)?

- 10 Points: You and your ally review your results weekly, enforce a "carrot/stick," and adjust.
- 7 Points: You and your ally review your results monthly and sometimes enforce "carrot/stick."
- 4 Points: You and your ally review your results quarterly.
- 0 Points: All else.

POINTS: _____

You know your number one Mindset Strength (Competitive Advantage):

- 10 points. Otherwise: 0 points.

POINTS: _____

You know your number one Mindset Weakness (Weak Link):

- 10 points. Otherwise: 0 points.

POINTS: _____

You know your number one Mindset Opportunity (Target):

- 10 points. Otherwise: 0 points.

POINTS: _____

You know your number one Mindset Threat (Enemy):

- 10 points. Otherwise: 0 points.

POINTS: _____

TOTAL POINTS: _____

OVERALL AVERAGE (TOTAL POINTS / 14) _____

This is the same process for your Knowledge Block. It is imperative to develop an elite Mindset. It is also imperative to develop a mastery of your sport. This is the Knowledge Block. The following set of questions only pertain to your Knowledge of certain things. There will be some redundancy with each section of questions with other Blocks. For example, you may have a mentor who helps you with more than one Inch Block. He may help you with your Mindset, Knowledge, and dealing with Teammates. That is perfectly acceptable. Simply answer the questions as best you can and tally your score.

<u>KNOWLEDGE</u>

Playbook (Points are doubled here because of their significance.)

- 20 Points: You know your critical skills, your position's duties, your unit's duties, your offense's or defense's duties, and your opponents' duties perfectly.
- 16 Points: You know all skills and duties for your position, unit, and your offense or defense.

- 14 Points: You know all skills and duties for your position and unit.
- 12 Points: You know all skills and duties for your position.
- 0 Points: You do not know your position skills and duties perfectly.

POINTS: _____

Life

- 10 Points: You have a plan and process to manage your critical life skills now and in the future for you to perform at your best in your sport.
- 7 Points: You are getting by day-to-day, and it affects your play.
- 2 Points: Your environment (clutter, cleanliness, paying bills, etc.) at home is in disarray.
- 0 Points: All else.

POINTS: _____

Kaizen

- 10 Points: You have a process for improving and adhere to it without fail.
- 8 Points: You mostly have a process and adhere to it.
- 5 Points: You occasionally have a process and adhere to it.
- 0 Points: All else.

POINTS: _____

Knowledge Mentor

- 10 Points: You have one and connect weekly.
- 8 Points: You have one and connect monthly.
- 5 Points: You have one and connect quarterly.
- 0 Points: All else.

POINTS: _____

How effectively are you working with a Knowledge accountability ally (or allies)?

- 10 Points: You and your ally review your results weekly, enforce a "carrot/stick," and adjust.
- 7 Points: You and your ally review your results monthly and sometimes enforce "carrot/stick."
- 4 Points: You and your ally review your results quarterly.
- 0 Points: All else.

POINTS: _____

You know your number one Knowledge Strength (Competitive Advantage):

- 10 points. Otherwise: 0 points.

POINTS: _____

You know your number one Knowledge Weakness (Weak Link):

- 10 points. Otherwise: 0 points.

POINTS: _____

You know your number one Knowledge Opportunity (Target):

- 10 points. Otherwise: 0 points.

POINTS: _____

You know your number one Knowledge Threat (Enemy):

- 10 points. Otherwise: 0 points.

POINTS: _____

TOTAL POINTS: _____

OVERALL AVERAGE (TOTAL POINTS / 10) _____

Your Teammates are the third Block pertaining to your head. This Block assesses your ability to work well with others. All your relationships make an impact on your level of play. Do not undervalue or underestimate the importance of everyone around you. It matters.

<u>TEAMMATES</u>

Players

- 10 Points: You are a captain of your team.
- 7 Points: You respect your Teammates, and they respect you. You work well with everyone and help get them better.
- 4 Points: You get your job done well and don't cause problems on your team. You mostly focus on yourself and not others.

POINTS: _____

Coaches

- 10 Points: You are the first one at the facility, last to leave, leader of your team, inform coaches, act as the "pulse of the team," are positive and upbeat, Relentless, and tough all the time.
- 8 Points: You mostly perform the duties listed above.
- 6 Points: You sometimes perform the duties listed above.
- 4 Points: You rarely perform the duties listed above.
- 0 Points: All else.

POINTS: _____

Professional Groups (teachers, trainers, medical staff, janitors, etc.)

- 10 Points: You are always respectful and professional, positive, supportive, and helpful.
- 8 points: You are mostly the qualities listed.
- 6 Points: You are sometimes the qualities listed.
- 4 Points: You are rarely the qualities listed.
- 0 Points: All else.

POINTS: _____

Kaizen

- 10 Points: You have a process for improving and adhere to it without fail.
- 8 Points: You mostly have a process and adhere to it.
- 5 Points: You occasionally have a process and adhere to it.
- 0 Points: All else.

POINTS: _____

Teammate Mentor

- 10 Points: You have one and connect weekly.
- 8 Points: You have one and connect monthly.
- 5 Points: You have one and connect quarterly.
- 0 Points: All else

POINTS: _____

How effectively are you working with a Teammate accountability ally (or allies)?

- 10 Points: You and your ally review your results weekly, enforce a "carrot/stick," and adjust.
- 7 Points: You and your ally review your results monthly and sometimes enforce "carrot/stick."
- 4 Points: You and your ally review your results quarterly.
- 0 Points: All else

POINTS: _____

You know your number one Teammate Strength (Competitive Advantage):

- 10 points. Otherwise: 0 points.

POINTS: _____

You know your number one Teammate Weakness (Weak Link):

- 10 points. Otherwise: 0 points.

POINTS: _____

You know your number one Teammate Opportunity (Target):

- 10 points. Otherwise: 0 points.

POINTS: _____

You know your number one Teammate Threat (Enemy):

- 10 points. Otherwise: 0 points.

POINTS: _____

TOTAL POINTS: _____

OVERALL AVERAGE (TOTAL POINTS /10) _____

This next section can be challenging to quantify the data. Your answers will require more estimations than normal. Information is not readily available. However, at times the data is available. Example: The NFL Combine publishes the year's results annually. There is historical data available as well. You will need the input from a strength and conditioning coach to give you a range of values or best guesses. You must find a coach if you don't have one.

<u>TRAINING</u>

Strength

- 10 Points: You are in the top 10 percent (in strength) at your position nationwide.
- 8 Points: You are in the top 10 percent in your conference.
- 6 Points: You are in the top 10 percent of your position group on team.
- 4 Points: You are in the top 20 percent of your position group on the team.

- 2 Points: You are in the top 50 percent of your position group on the team.
- 0 Points: All else.

POINTS: _____

Fastest and Most Powerful

- 10 Points: You are in the top 10 percent (in speed and power) at your position nationwide.
- 8 Points: You are in the top 10 percent in your conference.
- 6 Points: You are in the top 10 percent of your position group on the team.
- 4 Points: You are in the top 20 percent of your position group on the team.
- 2 Points: You are in the top 50 percent of your position group on the team.
- 0 Points: All else.

POINTS: _____

Stamina

- 10 Points: You are in the top 10 percent (in stamina) at your position nationwide.
- 8 Points: You are in the top 10 percent in your conference.
- 6 Points: You are in the top 10 percent of your position group on the team.
- 4 Points: You are in the top 20 percent of your position group on the team.

- 2 Points: You are in the top 50 percent of your position group on the team.
- 0 Points: All else.

POINTS: _____

Resiliency (You're the toughest.)

- 10 Points: You are in the top 10 percent (in resiliency) at your position nationwide.
- 8 Points: You are in the top 10 percent in your conference.
- 6 Points: You are in the top 10 percent of your position group on the team.
- 4 Points: You are in the top 20 percent of your position group on the team.
- 2 Points: You are in the top 50 percent of your position group on the team.
- 0 Points: All else.

POINTS: _____

Offseason

- 10 Points: You put in the most work of anyone on your team (in the gym and on the field, doing everything physical to improve).
- 8 Points: You are in the top ten people on your team for putting in the most work.
- 6 Points: You put in the most work of anyone in your position group.
- 0 Points: All else.

POINTS: _____

In-season

- 10 Points: You put in the most work of anyone on your team (in the gym and on the field, doing everything physical to improve).
- 8 Points: You are in the top ten people on your team for putting in the most work.
- 6 Points: You put in the most work of anyone in your position group.
- 0 Points: All else.

POINTS: _____

Kaizen

- 10 Points: You have a process for improving and adhere to it without fail.
- 8 Points: You mostly have a process and adhere to it.
- 5 Points: You occasionally have a process and adhere to it.
- 0 Points: All else.

POINTS: _____

Training Mentor

- 10 Points: You have one and connect weekly.
- 8 Points: You have one and connect monthly.
- 5 Points: You have one and connect quarterly.
- 0 Points: All else.

POINTS: _____

How effectively are you working with a Training accountability ally (or allies)?

- 10 Points: You and your ally review your results weekly, enforce a "carrot/stick," and adjust.
- 7 Points: You and your ally review your results monthly and sometimes enforce "carrot/stick."
- 4 Points: You and your ally review your results quarterly.
- 0 Points: All else.

POINTS: _____

You know your number one Training Strength (Competitive Advantage):

- 10 points. Otherwise: 0 points.

POINTS: _____

You know your number one Training Weakness (Weak Link):

- 10 points. Otherwise: 0 points.

POINTS: _____

You know your number one Training Opportunity (Target):

- 10 points. Otherwise: 0 points.

POINTS: _____

You know your number one Training Threat (Enemy):

- 10 points. Otherwise: 0 points.

POINTS: _____

TOTAL POINTS: _____

OVERALL AVERAGE (TOTAL POINTS /13) _____

Next, let's see where you stack up with your Nutrition. In sports and most things, results are what matters most. Certain athletes won't need any help with Nutrition. Other athletes will struggle mightily with it. Ultimately, what you eat will affect your results dramatically. Be diligent.

NUTRITION

Body Fat

- 10 Points: You are in the top 10 percent (in body fat) at your position nationwide.
- 8 Points: You are in the top 10 percent in your conference.
- 6 Points: You are in the top 10 percent of your position group on team.
- 4 Points: You are in the top 20 percent of your position group on the team.

- 2 Points: You are in the top 50 percent of your position group on the team.
- 0 Points: All else.

POINTS: _____

Protein, Creatine, and Supplements

- 10 Points: You have a process to perfect performance and adhere to it always.
- 8 Points: You mostly have a process and adhere to it.
- 6 Points: You sometimes have a process and adhere to it.
- 4 Points: You rarely have a process and adhere to it.
- 0 Points: All else.

POINTS: _____

Offseason Total Nutrition Plan

- 10 Points: You have a process to perfect performance and adhere to it always.
- 8 Points: You mostly have a process and adhere to it.
- 6 Points: You sometimes have a process and adhere to it.
- 4 Points: You rarely have a process and adhere to it.
- 0 Points: All else.

POINTS: _____

In-season Home Games

- 10 Points: You have a process to perfect performance and adhere to it always.
- 8 Points: You mostly have a process and adhere to it.
- 6 Points: You sometimes have a process and adhere to it.
- 4 Points: You rarely have a process and adhere to it.
- 0 Points: All else.

POINTS: _____

In-season Away Games

- 10 Points: You have a process to perfect performance and adhere to it always.
- 8 Points: You mostly have a process and adhere to it.
- 6 Points: You sometimes have a process and adhere to it.
- 4 Points: You rarely have a process and adhere to it.
- 0 Points: All else.

POINTS: _____

Kaizen

- 10 Points: You have a process for improving and adhere to it without fail.
- 8 Points: You mostly have a process and adhere to it.
- 5 Points: You occasionally have a process and adhere to it.
- 0 Points: All else.

POINTS: _____

Nutrition Mentor

- 10 Points: You have one and connect weekly.
- 8 Points: You have one and connect monthly.
- 5 Points: You have one and connect quarterly.
- 0 Points: All else.

POINTS: _____

How effectively are you working with a Nutrition accountability ally (or allies)?

- 10 Points: You and your ally review your results weekly, enforce a "carrot/stick," and adjust.
- 7 Points: You and your ally review your results monthly and sometimes enforce "carrot/stick."
- 4 Points: You and your ally review your results quarterly.
- 0 Points: All else.

POINTS: _____

You know your number one Nutrition Strength (Competitive Advantage):

- 10 points. Otherwise: 0 points.

POINTS: _____

You know your number one Nutrition Weakness (Weak Link):

- 10 points. Otherwise: 0 points.

POINTS: _____

You know your number one Nutrition Opportunity (Target):

- 10 points. Otherwise: 0 points.

POINTS: _____

You know your number one Nutrition Threat (Enemy):

- 10 points. Otherwise: 0 points.

POINTS: _____

TOTAL POINTS: _____

OVERALL AVERAGE (TOTAL POINTS /12) _____

RECOVERY

Injuries

- 10 Points: No major injuries for the year and missed no reps in games and practice.
- 8 Points: Hurt but missed no reps in games.
- 6 Points: Missed 20 percent of the games and practice reps.
- 4 Points: Missed 40 percent of game and practice reps.
- 0 Points: Missed more than half of the season.

POINTS: _____

Resting and Sleep Process

- 10 Points: You have a process to perfect performance and adhere to it always.
- 8 Points: You mostly have a process and adhere to it.
- 6 Points: You sometimes have a process and adhere to it.
- 4 Points: You rarely have a process and adhere to it.
- 0 Points: All else.

POINTS: _____

Treatments

- 10 Points: You have a process to perfect performance and adhere to it always.
- 8 Points: You mostly have a process and adhere to it.
- 6 Points: You sometimes have a process and adhere to it.
- 4 Points: You rarely have a process and adhere to it.
- 0 Points: All else.

POINTS: _____

Breathing and Meditation

- 10 Points: You have a process to perfect performance and adhere to it always.
- 8 Points: You mostly have a process and adhere to it.
- 6 Points: You sometimes have a process and adhere to it.
- 4 Points: You rarely have a process and adhere to it.
- 0 Points: All else.

POINTS: _____

Traveling

- 10 Points: You have a process to perfect performance and adhere to it always.
- 8 Points: You mostly have a process and adhere to it.
- 6 Points: You sometimes have a process and adhere to it.
- 4 Points: You rarely have a process and adhere to it.
- 0 Points: All else.

POINTS: _____

Kaizen

- 10 Points: You have a process for improving and adhere to it without fail.
- 8 Points: You mostly have a process and adhere to it.
- 5 Points: You occasionally have a process and adhere to it.
- 0 Points: All else.

POINTS: _____

Recovery Mentor

- 10 Points: You have one and connect weekly.
- 8 Points: You have one and connect monthly.
- 5 Points: You have one and connect quarterly.
- 0 Points: All else.

POINTS: _____

How effectively are you working with a Recovery accountability ally (or allies)?

- 10 Points: You and your ally review your results weekly, enforce a "carrot/stick," and adjust.
- 7 Points: You and your ally review your results monthly and sometimes enforce "carrot/stick."
- 4 Points: You and your ally review your results quarterly.
- 0 Points: All else.

POINTS: _____

You know your number one Recovery Strength (Competitive Advantage):

- 10 points. Otherwise: 0 points.

POINTS: _____

You know your number one Recovery Weakness (Weak Link):

- 10 points. Otherwise: 0 points.

POINTS: _____

You know your number one Recovery Opportunity (Target):

- 10 points. Otherwise: 0 points.

POINTS: _____

You know your number one Recovery Threat (Enemy):

- 10 points. Otherwise: 0 points.

POINTS: _____

TOTAL POINTS: _____

OVERALL AVERAGE (TOTAL POINTS /12) _____

TOTAL OF THE 7 AVERAGES: _____

INCHES AVERAGE (TOTAL OF 7 AVERAGES / 7) _____

Here is how I look at the overall average. Remember, there are different levels of athletes. Pretenders are the losers that clearly don't have it. They have next to no Discipline. They are going nowhere. . . currently. But any Pretender can turn on a dime and elevate himself the next day. I've seen it many times. This is how we are looking at the averages:

- Pretenders: 0–3. It's decision time here. Either quit and look elsewhere or get it together and commit. Now.
- 5: Minimum. This only gets you 50 percent of the way. Think about that. Check yourself and see if I'm off on this. Do you think you're going pro or far in college or the pros with a score of 5? Nope.
- 6: College Scholarship. Depending on the sport, you're one of the best on your team, conference, and state. Example: For football, about 7 percent of players get to play at either D1, D2,

D3, D1-AA, and NAIA. All combined, that's 7 percent of high school players. All but D3 can get college money.

- 7: You're a college starter. Period.
- 8: College All-American. Talent and the team you're on could (rarely) carry you to this level. But it's so unlikely that betting on that approach is embarrassing. Don't gamble. Work your ass off instead.
- 9: Pro. And Pro at a high level. What's that look like, statistically? Take football again. 7 percent play in college. 1.8 percent of those go pro. There are seven rounds in the draft, multiplied by thirty-two teams. The number divided by the 125 D1 teams (not even adding those that make it from lower levels) times the typical hundred-man roster leaves 1.8 percent. You are legit at this level. So far, your chance is 7 percent × 1.8 percent = 0.00126. Or 0.126 percent.
- 10: The Statue. You have a bust in the Hall of Fame in Canton. There are thirty-two teams with fifty-three-man rosters. The HOF takes eight per year, at most. That means that 0.47 percent make it each year. Half a percent makes it each year. But wait—this does not include all the retired players who are eligible for the HOF. That number is much larger. But for our example 7 percent play in college, 1.8 percent go pro, and 0.47 percent make it to the Hall. What does that look like for you? It's 0.059 percent. That is about half of a hundredth of a percent (it's actually much harder than that). Read that about eighty-seven more times to let it sink in.

<u>Scan the following QR code</u> or visit: https://athlete-builder.com to access and download this assessment and other resources (free nutrition resources and free workout programs).

CHAPTER 12

MINDSET - DECISIONS

*"*M*ental toughness is to the physical as four is to one."*
– Bobby Knight

This is the one. This is it. Each Inch Block is a "must." Each is critical for success. Some sections can be "faked" longer than other sections. But all must be sound, strengthened, and optimized. But this section is the one. I get asked all the time, "What's the one thing I need to do to win?" I just shake my head. It's so sad, really. There is never just one thing. Good Lord. Has life ever been that easy to distill down to one thing? No. What a simple-minded approach. And it's fatal. In this case it's still true. There is *not* just one thing. However, of the six Blocks to Inches, the Mindset pillar is the one thing. Of course, this pillar has a thousand things to work on. It's not just one thing here. But it's obvious, right? How you think determines what you do. And what you do is all that matters. The brain thinks, feels, assesses, determines, decides, and then moves the body forward. Everything is mental. Everything. We are working to tame, influence, and control our brains. We fight not to be slaves to emotion. So, you need to figure this part out. Now. Get your mind right and win. If you don't, you'll lose. Or worse. . . give up.

Decide. Choose. Pick. Then go!

Change

There are no absolutes. There are also laws to follow. So, which is it? You know the answer: It depends. People don't change. Absolute? No. People do change. The problem is that it's so rare that people change in a meaningful way that it makes sense to say, "People don't change." Why? Because typically they don't. That means you typically won't either. Here's also an unfortunate byproduct: People's perception of you won't change. Absolute? No. People change their minds. It just takes a ton of evidence. That's why first impressions are critical.

There are two ways people change. Option 1: Something cathartic must occur. What does that mean? It means something overwhelming and life-changing must happen. The event is so impactful that you change your identity and behavior at once.

Hypothetical example: You're a huge drinker. One day, you crash your car coming home from a party. The next day you decide never to drink again. You get help and make life changes. And it's done. You're a new person when it comes to drinking.

Personal example: I went through a divorce in 2007–2008. I did things wrong and sucked at being a husband. One thing that stuck out was that I would hold ideas and feelings in. I'd bottle them up and fake things. I wasn't as authentic as I had to be to live a life I wanted. A divorce can change you if you want. And it did for me. I'm still miles away from being perfect. But I consciously strive to be authentic and real with everyone. People will get and understand the real me.

Option 2: You want to change and take massive action. How much is massive? It's more action than what you think you can do and more action than most want to do initially. Unless you really want to change. You must change. In this case, the work is fun because you want it. This is the route you are taking now with *Inches*. You are systematically and Relentlessly striving and grinding each day. You are on a special path. And that path will lead you to your highest levels as an athlete. It will only occur if you work at it every day. For the greatest athletes of all time, it becomes an obsession.

Change = Opportunity. Absolute? It depends. For me? Yes. It's an absolute. I believe it and work that way. I know and believe what I just wrote in the last five paragraphs above. (Go back and reread them.) So, I know that most, not all, hate and don't want to change. If I take the approach that it's an opportunity, then I'll adapt and evolve faster than those dragging their feet and resisting it. While others are complaining, I am advancing. I'm getting an edge. They are staying stagnant or worse, regressing. I'm winning and moving forward. And I'll win because of it. So. Can. You!

Which Level Are You?

I categorized people in different levels of sporting greatness at the end of the Assessment Test. This is a refresher if you skipped it or forgot. There are the **Pretenders.** If you're reading this book and training to play in college or the pros, then the Pretenders don't even count. They aren't in the discussion. Depending on your sport, between 3 percent and 13 percent move from high school to college. You can Google any number of studies to find similar data. Playing at the D1 level means you're most likely in the top 2 percent or less. The Pretenders don't make it to that level. What does that mean for you? Simple. Be the top one or two players on your team, and you'll have a solid chance to advance.

Next level is the **College Athlete.** That's obvious, right? The difference here is between the D1, D2, D3, D1-AA, and NAIA levels of athlete. What does that look like, statistically. Again, simple. Qualify as an All-State candidate, and you have a good shot at the D1, D2 level. (Note: Simple ≠ Easy.)

Pro Athlete? Again, simple. Be the top player on your team is a good start. All-conference and All-American or more obvious milestones indicate that you can play in the pros. You'll need to be a significant impact player. The means other teams must game-plan around you. And if the pros see you are that level of player in college, then you've got a shot at your first pro contract.

Then there is **The Statue.** This would equate to Tim Grover's "Cleaner" level of comparison. The Statue is the one with his own plaque or bust or likeness in the Hall of Fame. This is the Payton Manning outside Indy's stadium and Michael Jordan outside Chicago's. At the Pro Football Hall of Fame in Canton, Ohio, there are busts of all its members. But there is only one full-size statue greeting people at its doors. It's Jim Thorpe. It's the statue of the Marines raising the flag at Iwo Jima as portrayed in Arlington National Cemetery. It's Abe Lincoln's and Martin Luther King's enormous likenesses in Washington, DC. It is era-changing, civilization-changing, sports-changing greatness.

Decide. Which are you? Now, which are you, today? Good chance you're not Dr. Martin Luther King today. At a young age, Martin King wasn't Dr. Martin King either. But he was on his path to greatness. This brings us back to you, today. Which are you today? Be honest with yourself (*Temet nosce.* Know thyself.) Are you a Pretender today? Pro athlete today? Next, what will you be? Today, tomorrow, in five years, in thirty years? You must choose. Choose the path you want to be on. Pretender. College athlete. Pro athlete. Or the Statue.

Stop what you're doing. Close your eyes and be still. Breathe deeply for five minutes. Any thought that enters your mind must leave. Inhale thoughts through your nose. And send them out through your mouth. Repeat until your mind is blank. Then ask yourself: Which will you be? At your core, you must know. When you know, stand up. Go to the bathroom and stare in the mirror. Look at that face. "See" your mind. Think. Think deeply. Decide. What are you now? And what will you be? Not tomorrow, but once you turn away from the mirror. . . which path *must* you be on? It's the path you *are* on once you turn away. Choose now. Pick. Decide.

Great news. This is one of the few big decisions you must make. The next big one is when you decide to advance or regress to the nearest level.

Otherwise, the hard decisions are over. The other decisions are simple, tactical ones that improve performance. What people don't understand is that when you are struggling in high school and decide to play in college, most other decisions get taken away. They are gone. For good. This decision gives you only a few things to do and takes away everything else.

Ultimately, the ability to decide is an illusion. Example: You decide to enter the US Navy. You sign the papers, show up at MEPS for processing. Then you start basic training (i.e., boot camp). The next morning, boot camp starts at 05:00. You don't get to decide if you get out of bed the next morning to arrive to your first task before 05:00. The choice is gone. It was made. You must arrive and do what's instructed.

The same is true here with you. Get that through your head. You don't get to play on Sundays in the NFL without doing the extra treatments to keep your body healthy during your final college season. You don't really get to skip out on treatments during the years before. Certain things are now requirements. They are not suggestions. If you think they are, you've lost. You won't last. Turn that mindset around now. If you don't, then you'll be done a lot sooner than you like.

Personal example: Candy Bars. In 1986, I was living in Euclid, Ohio (a suburb of Cleveland) in a very modest house with my family. I was twelve years old and it was the first year my family had enough money or interest for me to play little league baseball. Baseball started at age seven and ended at twelve. But for me, it started at twelve. One requirement to play was that I sell one box of thirty candy bars at $1/bar. I needed to turn the money in to the manager so I could earn a uniform. It was non-negotiable. I did it quickly the first couple nights and was done. Cool.

The manager, a great guy named Dave Anderson, told me that if I sold more, then I could get some prizes. "Like what?" I asked. Well, it turned out that a new Nintendo was one of the prizes. I had asked for one the prior December for my birthday or Christmas. It was $99 at the time, a lot of money for us. And I didn't receive one. "How many boxes must I sell?" I asked. The answer was easy: Thirty-six. That's thirty-six boxes of thirty bars. That's 1,080 bars if you're doing the math.

Long story short, I sold them all. I simply rode my bike or got dropped off in different neighborhoods each day and went door-to-door. I sold more on weekends. Problem solved. I received my Nintendo and started playing Super Mario Brothers immediately. Sounds simple enough, right? It depends. (Most life questions have the same answer.) Yes, I had a straightforward opportunity and plan: Sell 1,080 bars. Of course, not everyone was home when I knocked on the door, and not everyone bought a bar when I asked. Then there were times when a family would buy five or six bars. I know this for sure: I had to ask a lot more than 1,080 times if someone wanted a candy bar. As "good" as I was, my close rate was not 100 percent.

It's not an amazing story. It's simple. I wanted Q. It cost P. If I did P, then I got Q. I decided and then went to work. You'll see a similar theme throughout this book with my habits and results. To quote Trevor Moawad's book title, *It Takes What It Takes*. Deciding is the hard part. Once you do, look out! Then simply go all in and over-execute until you win. Repeat.

Personal example: College Pro Painters. My parents divorced long ago, when I was two years old. My father wrote in the divorce decree that he'd pay for my college. As I was choosing schools, he said I could go to any school that would accept me. University of Cincinnati, University of Michigan, and Purdue accepted me for engineering. I chose Purdue. Fast forward, it was now late in 1994. I was in my third semester at Purdue University. It was out-of-state tuition for me, which meant the cost for school was $17,000 a year. I called my dad because a bill wasn't paid. He told me he was out of money. No notice. No forewarning. Typical of him. He was a horrible communicator, among other things.

Soon after, I was home for Christmas break, and I received a general solicitation in the mail to apply with College Pro Painters (CPP) and become a franchisee. (Jesus was looking out for me again.) I needed a bunch of money after the spring semester debt I was about to take on, and I knew more debt was coming with the future years of college left. I investigated CPP further. It was going to be a mountain of work for some twenty-year-old to start a business and run it well enough to cover my expenses. To make $17,000+ in a summer is quite a bit. It came down to this: I needed X, and it cost Y. It wasn't that I'd "like" to have X. Or "wouldn't it be sweet" if I got X? No. I *must* have X. I had to decide. To commit. And then execute.

I said "yes" and took the job. That meant that during the Spring semester, I went through training in Indianapolis on weekends. I didn't have a car yet, so I had to borrow a ride each time. Then I spent all spring break estimating houses to be painting jobs. Once classes ended, I started training the crews I recently hired, and we started painting houses. There were a lot of houses. I ended up doing commercial work, too. Summer ended, and I kept painting crews. I would leave a job site in my paint clothes, head to class at Purdue, and then go back to the site afterward. By fall break, I was done painting. The first year resulted in $69,000 in revenue and about $13,000 in profit for tuition. I was only a little short, which meant a much smaller loan. I was rookie of the year for College Pro in Indiana, which landed me a free trip to Florida that winter. Boom! The next two years were better. In the end, I ended up with less than one full year of student loans after nine semesters at Purdue and my degree in Business Management. (Engineering didn't stick. But that's a story for a different section of the book.)

The point is to decide. Decide like your life depends on it because it does. I'm not joking. It wasn't literally life or death. My life didn't depend on it that way. But the direction my life will take always depends on my decisions. In addition, who you are and who you become depend on your decisions. It is so liberating. You will feel so free once you decide and have clarity. The stressors are changed because you're no longer wondering "would I, should I, could I." Decide. Move forward.

This is the make-or-break point of the book. This is the make-or-break point of view. If you decide to "burn the boats" (Cortés and his ships. . . another story) and commit to your highest level or even a higher level of "you," then keep moving forward with what to do next. If you can't or won't decide, good luck. It's immensely harder. So, my advice if you're on the fence is this: Decide to be a little better the rest of to-day. That's it. The rest of today. What is one thing you can do today to advance yourself a little? Do that. Then keep progressing with that path you're on here. Most will say "fake it until you make it." Well, what the hell does that mean? What's the process for that? It's okay. Most like to use catch phrases to motivate. I do too. But more importantly, I'll give you steps and a process to do it. Let's keep moving forward.

Next, ask yourself what's holding you back from committing? I'm sure you have some lies as to why you allegedly can't do something. You read the sentence, so I know your mind went there and you already have some thoughts on why you're unable to advance. They are all lies. It's okay. Write them down now. Answer me!

What are your limiting beliefs? Why can't you win? Why can't you advance? What's holding you back? Let's address this next. If we don't, we're stuck. And that's unacceptable. Because we. Must. Move. For-ward.

CHAPTER 13

MINDSET - LIMITING BELIEFS

Did you do the work at the end of the last section? Were you honest? I mean stop-what-you're-doing, look-in-the-mirror honest? Do you have your list now? All right, which one is the big one? What's the main "reason" you "can't" do something? Do you have that one?

Look in the mirror and say it out loud. "I can't." Say it again. Again. Or honestly, it might be "I'm afraid of. . . because. . . ." Say that three times. Do it.

Examples:

- I could never play in college. Or I could never play in the pros. I'm not good enough.
- I'm not fast enough.
- The coach hates me, and I don't get enough playing time.
- I'm afraid to ask the coach about this. I could never discuss this with a coach.
- It's not that I'm afraid of doing extra work. I'm afraid I may do it, and it won't matter. The coach won't notice. I still won't improve. I still won't get more playing time.
- My peers will tease me for trying hard. It's even a common term, a "try hard."

- Friends, family, or teammates will ridicule me for saying I want to play in college or play pro.

On a deep psychological level, it's going to be this: I'm afraid to try to do this because I could fail. And if I fail, then I'll look weak and less desirable. And if I appear weak and less desirable, then no one will like me. And people won't want to hang around with me. The final belief becomes "My family and friends will abandon me. I'll end up alone." That's the main fear for most. Well, it's how the fear progresses. It's typically not on a fully conscious level but more of a subconscious level. It's different for everyone.

Your fears are always your biggest opponent. Forever. It wages war in your head. Other times, it isn't fear at all but other thoughts and habits. Again, it's how you are thinking. It's what you're thinking about. It's your real and imagined beliefs. God, aren't you sick of being held down by your thoughts? How can you stand it? Don't you just get sick to your stomach knowing you're in your own way? Check out these lies you may have told yourself in the past. I know I did at least once in my life:

How about this lie? "I'm not good enough. I will never be good enough. I can't manage the workload."

How about this sly, subtle lie? "I am good enough right here at this level. I don't need to keep working this hard. I should take some time off. I'm too obsessed and out of control. I should just take it easy from here; I deserve it."

Here is one of the worst destructive paths: "I think I tried enough. The coach or boss doesn't see it because I'm not his favorite. I could never break through. I should just quit now."

Goodness! Shut up! Just find your next target and move forward. There is no stopping where you're on this path. The targets are not the end or the destination. The journey and the process are the destination. Love the grind and you'll keep going every day. *(Real note: it's 6/3/23 and I'm in the editing stage of this book. It's 6:47 a.m. local Vancouver, Canada time. I am on a family vacation and will do a hike this morning before boarding a boat later. But the editing must be done by my target date so I can publish this book. It takes what it takes.)*

Consider *Indiana Jones and the Quest for the Holy Grail.* It's an amazing series, and Harrison Ford is legendary in it. This film was the third installment, and it didn't disappoint. Near the end of the film, Ford's character, Indiana Jones, must pass three tests to find the Holy Grail. The grail, once filled with holy water, will supply a magic elixir that will cure the sick or dying. To make matters worse, Jones's father has been captured by a Nazi and is dying from a wound. On the third challenge, the leap of faith, Jones exits a tunnel and looks across a huge cavern of more than thirty feet. On the other side is the doorway to the grail. It's an impossible leap for anyone. He looks around, seeing only rock and granite everywhere. It surrounds his cave exit. It makes up the entirety of the cavern. And it's also what creates the passageway across the cavern. He knows it is unequivocally impossible.

His father is dying. Nonetheless, his map and book instruct him to make his "leap of faith" from this exact point. The prior steps worked out as planned. But how could this one? You see it on his face. It's complete denial. It says it's impossible. He has no choice, however. Why? He made his choice earlier that he would do everything to save his father.

Next, with his hand over his heart, he clutches his book and map. You see the resolve wash over his face as he accepts his decision amid his uncertainty. He stretches out his foot and pauses. Then he does all he can do; he leans forward and takes a step.

Magically, it lands and catches hold on solid footing! How? Impossible? He takes a second step. Then he looks around. There's a bridge he couldn't see before. The camouflaged bridge blends in with the rock surroundings. It looks identical. He simply didn't recognize it. He takes another step and then another, and even more steps. He's walking across the bridge. You watch the realization on his face. Confidence increases with every step. Now he's happy as he makes his way across the bridge to the next entrance. Once there, he throws a handful of pebbles and sand across the bridge so he and others can see the path as well.

Once the possible occurred, there was a reminder that it could occur again.

He and you must take that step and move forward.

Is it that simple? You bet it is. No one said it was easy, but it is that simple. Look. There is almost nothing new and profound in the world in terms of human nature and behavior. "The only thing new in the world is the history we do not know," said Harry Truman.

If you can and choose to, then take a step and move forward. The end. Move on.

If you are currently unable and struggling, then implement this process. At any point along the way in the process, it will still come back to the same thing. You'll have to take a step and move forward. But this will help get you unstuck and able to progress:

- Say the fear aloud three times if you haven't already.
- Write it down.
- Share it with your accountability ally.

It should start to sink in that what you're saying and writing is silly and unreasonable. It will begin to appear to be a bit ridiculous. Next:

- Take ten deep breaths and repeat the above process. That's right. Breathing changes your physiology and your psyche. Use it to calm yourself down and repeat.
- Now check your "Why." This equation must hold true: Why > Fear or Concern. If your "Why" wins the battle, great. Now take a step and move forward. This must happen. Take action.
- Still stuck? Now write out all the positives and negatives to what moving forward entails. You see what we are doing here? We are working to take the emotion out of the situation because it is hurting you. You're breaking down and losing the Mindset battle. We must get your mind to shut the hell up and listen. Now think!

- Not there? Write out the next three steps and name the critical one. Good. Now step forward.
- At this point, have you asked for help? If you can't or won't progress alone, then you must get help and move forward that way. Get ahold of me. Or find another coach. Find someone. But make sure you pick someone that will get movement out of you. That's when people come to me. I will demand movement and results, so don't ask me unless you're all in.
- You will know you are winning when you are taking action.

If you won't move forward, there isn't much more for us to do. If you're ready, then let's progress. Design your process. Process is king. It isn't negotiable. Process leads to a small win. It gives you the belief that you can improve because you see it. Then confidence must go up. Why? Because you saw and felt you could do it. Then you did it. Then you know! Then what? Refine and evolve your process. Take another step on your leap of faith journey. Improve a little more. Build more confidence. Improve again. Repeat until you win it all or can no longer do it.

CHAPTER 14

MINDSET - BRAINWASHING

Confidence versus cockiness. You know the difference. You can see it; shoot, you can smell it sometimes. Well, confidence only comes from reps. Cockiness is the weak-minded talking loudly and boldly as a smoke screen. It's all he has left, and he knows it. So his fear is coming through, and he's masking it with false bravado. It's not real and therefore not sustainable.

I once asked my stepdaughter, Lauren, to look at two of the cops who train in my gym, Mikey and Chris. Both are exceptional and dear friends. Mikey is forty-seven years old and a K9 cop. Chris, a lieutenant, is older, closer to retiring. Mikey is a little more outgoing, with a crazy, fun personality. Chris is fun too, but a little more reserved. I asked Lauren one day, "Who do you want on your team in a fight?"

She quickly responded, "Mikey." I asked why. "He's younger, not as banged up as Chris, has a dog on his team. I think he'd win." And to be clear, Mikey is all those things and a true badass with no fear.

Then I said, "Well, Chris is a former Army Ranger. Mikey is good at hand-to-hand combat, but Chris is the expert and teaches it. Mikey is great with his weapon, but Chris is the expert and teaches that as well." Chris is the James Bond who calmly walks into the room, smiles, and engages, but has a plan and method to kill everyone in it. That's confidence. And for the record, the current answer is "Both." You want both on your team. One personality is more outgoing than the other. Neither of them is a big talker, touting how good he is. They don't have to. And it's best to let everyone underestimate them.

How do you develop and improve confidence? The answer is reps. It's really the only answer. Let's look at Mohammad Ali. In February of 1964, he faced the heavyweight champion in boxing, Sonny Liston, for the first time. Ali was an 8:1 underdog. By the seventh round, Liston couldn't get off his stool in his corner and refused to reenter the ring to fight. The prior six rounds had been dominated by the underdog, and Liston wouldn't have any more of it. Ali won by TKO (Technical Knockout). The rematch in 1965 was worse for Liston. It was a first-round knockout. Over. Done. Next.

The interesting thing was that Ali had been talking about his future wins well before they occurred. Was that confidence for cockiness? Well, it depends. (The answer to most every question is "It depends.") Maybe Ali was supremely prepared. Maybe Ali just spoke more. Or maybe it's the preparation that leads to confidence. Speaking out and being loud may or may not be a smoke screen. Often it is, but there are no absolutes in life. Prepare for everything. In Ali's case, he was loud and brash but also supremely prepared. Train your Mindset to push yourself until you're the best in the six different Inch Blocks. Then you are supremely prepared. Push yourself to that point.

How could Ali be so confident? Think of it like this. How many games are in the NFL? Currently in 2022, there are seventeen games. How many hours are spent preparing outside the seventeen games? Hundreds and thousands! How fights did Ali have a year? It varied each year, but he fought in at least two and sometimes five fights a year. How much time was spent preparing? Hundreds and thousands of hours. Ali's confidence grew because he was obsessively and Relentlessly thorough in his preparation process. He knew what he could do, and what Liston could do before entering the ring. Remember Sun Tzu: "All wars are won before they are ever fought." As one last example of Ali's preparation, consider how critical core strength is for a fighter. (It's critical for all athletes. Critical.) Once, someone asked Ali how many sit-ups he did in a session. He responded he didn't know.

"How can that be, Ali?!" they asked.

He said, "I don't know. I only start counting the reps when they start hurting." If you're supremely prepared, you can play fast. You're confident. It takes that level of preparation at the highest level.

What does that have to do with brainwashing? The answer also aligns with the question "How do you develop confidence without the actual game-time reps?" Remember, there are only seventeen NFL games a year and for Ali a half-dozen fights per year or less. How can you have a belief before doing the actual deed? At the first stage, it's very rare to have that belief. A select few might truly believe in themselves fully, but c'mon. Really? No, it's rare. Not impossible, but rare. So, then what? Inches are the answer. Start your day and move forward toward your goal, your direction. And earn your confidence. Only your actions will enable your mind to know that you earned it. Most people are deathly afraid of public speaking. Well, what if you had to speak on your favorite topic? That's not so terrifying at all because you know the material. You're prepared. Conversely, what if you had a day to prepare to talk to a large crowd on the topic of cell regeneration after chemotherapy treatments? Answer: For almost everyone, it's panic! The difference is preparation. Always is, always will be.

Time to move forward and execute. We must pump your head full of the right Knowledge, emotions, and action items so it's ingrained in you. Here's how:

Brainwashing is the act of washing over your brain with a consistent set of ideas and information. You are systematically aligning your thinking with those ideas. Brainwashing can be a good, useful tool. It can also be a horrible, destructive tool. It can be a conscious or unconscious action as well. You already do it daily. You've been doing it your whole life. You went to school, where hopefully your teachers brainwashed you with useful knowledge. You're brainwashed in math year after year until you can improve and manage higher level problems. You're also brainwashed to learn history, science, social studies, etc. If you go to church, you're brainwashed with repeated messages about Christ, living a good and decent life, forgiveness, and other worthwhile themes. It can also be rat poison for yourself when you scroll endlessly on useless social media. Not only did you add a bit of cancer to your Mindset, but you also wasted a ton of time with negative brainwashing. So why not put it into action and create the Mindset you must have? Let's do that.

Here is an example of how I brainwash myself consistently:

I walk or hike or ruck march each morning (hike with a forty- to sixty-pound backpack on) daily. Nine times out of ten, I'm listening to something while doing so. I put on podcasts or YouTube videos of Eric Thomas, Inky Johnson, Jocko Willink, or David Goggins. Other times I'm listening to an educational audiobook. In that instance, I'm trying to learn how they speak, what their message might be, and what actions I can take to improve. I'm learning daily.

Or I'll pull up Joe Rogan and find a podcast with a guest on nutrition or sleeping better. If I'm looking for something specific to learn and improve, I will find others speaking on the same topic and listen to different viewpoints each morning for a week.

Other times, I'll listen to Ray Lewis, Michael Jordan, Kobe Bryant, or Tim Grover for their motivational talks. I select motivational speeches in the mornings. I'm looking to change my Mindset. Or I'm doing it to get excited and focused about a challenging task or training session that morning. I'm altering my Mindset deliberately based on what I need that morning. Either way, I'm pumping information into my head that I can use.

In each instance mentioned, I'm using Knowledge, motivational speeches, or even music to get my Mindset where it needs to be. There is still another method that is the complete opposite. There are a few mornings that I walk in complete silence. It enables me to dial in my thoughts to something specific. There is immense value in walking and thinking in silence as well. Do not discount that.

Next after I get home, I do two more things. I start my day with breakfast, usually a protein shake or Greek yogurt with a lot of fruit, and I do my devotional work. While I'm eating, I'm trying to be thankful with what I have and mindful that God gave it to me. The world is a hard place. We must strive to be our best versions of ourselves. I feel that God has called me to show people how to struggle and fight and kick and strive to be the best version of themselves. We must do this in honor of Him. That's my reminder to myself and my brainwashing process.

Next, I spend time downstairs in my office to read and journal. Usually, I must make a few quick notes on what was covered when I was listening during my walk. From there, I either spend fifteen minutes or half an hour reading or researching a topic I'm exploring, or I write down my own ideas and researching processes to help perfect those ideas. But usually, I have a book in my hand that I'm writing all over, dog-earring it so I can find the important pages, and taking copious notes so I can improve. There really are no innovative ideas out there. It's just the history we don't know or remember. That's what I'm doing now. I'm combining my life experiences and skills together with other experts to evolve. Then if I can share this with you in this book, a planner, or an app, then you can take everything from me and add your own ideas. Then you can further evolve the processes for others. And that is how the world turns and advances.

After working on my business for a couple of hours, I make sure I am "squared away" with the other tasks I have for that day, and I head to the gym to train. Once there, I pick one of three routes to combine brainwashing with my training. First, I may want or need to have music playing to distract me while I suffer through the session. Or I return to a Tony Robbins, David Goggins, or Navy SEAL montage to keep my mindset aggressive while I'm attacking a session. Or thirdly, I train in complete silence. Sometimes I like to be in my head while going through something. My little voice inside will say the craziest and purest things. I want to be able to hear it when he needs to speak something useful and meaningful.

That's a typical morning session of structured brainwashing for me. When I do it enough days in a row, I'm more motivated, focused, and driven. Helpful information and energy are pouring in, and I'm receiving help from it. It is improving my confidence in all areas. I'm training better. I get more done. I have more energy. I'm getting smarter. I'm accelerating my evolution deliberately. I'm advancing faster than others and much more than I was before. I'm winning!

Let's be clear, too. I don't do this much "content overload" every day. But I do it enough during the week that it helps me improve consistently.

Let's look at two processes for you to tackle next. Think about brainwashing yourself broadly or in general terms. Then think about doing the same thing very narrowly and specifically.

Broadly

Look at a typical physical training session for you. You're running for distance or have a weight-training session. You should have music that motivates or inspires. Hard, physical activity requires focus and a mild dose of adrenaline. Therefore, keep the music upbeat. (Again, not always. Sometimes you must self-motivate.)

Other mornings when I'm walking or training, I'll have David Goggins, Jocko Willink, or Kobe Bryant playing. The general topic could be motivational, about discipline or about suffering. The goal is to keep the same message embedded in my psyche throughout the session to penetrate to my subconscious. We want to develop the Sisu mindset.

Specifically

Whenever I attempt a new PR (Personal Record), there are only a handful of songs I listen to during the rep. The first isn't even a song.

It's the Haka by New Zealand's rugby team (All Blacks). It's a cultural tribal chant or incantation asking for prior souls and spirits of prior All Blacks. The team is asking for increased strength and grit to survive the next test. (Rugby refers to games or matches as tests. It's fitting, as it's a test of the teams' preparation, abilities, and execution.) Otherwise, I pick Kid Rock's "Bahwitdaba," "Bullets" by Creed, or any song from *Rocky*.

More specifically than the broad Sisu Mindset, I pull up a discussion on Kobe's Five Pillars of Success: Passionate, Relentless, Resilient, Fearless, and Obsessive. I'm looking for items that align with my Core Values and may introduce ones that I hadn't considered. This helps me expand my approach and general Mindset. It requires me to add or adjust habits. Naturally, performance will improve.

Here's the deal and the point: Spend time daily injecting useful knowledge, ideas, and mantras into your conscious and subconscious. Be specific. Be strategic. Be deliberate. Next, put those thoughts and newfound wisdom into practice. Pick two new habits. Track them for four to eight weeks and evaluate, change, and tweak. Once those habits are ingrained and perfected, it's time to elevate your game and do it again. Wash; rinse; repeat. The cycle never ends. Keep moving forward.

The brainwashing process will aid and improve your Mindset. First, it will help develop and instill confidence. You, the athlete, will start to believe in yourself because other, credible people are telling you to. They are telling you it's possible. You know why? Because it *is* possible. "Possible" is all you need. Then your only task is to find a way. Regardless, you will start to develop confidence before you have started earning any of the real repetitions that solidify confidence. Start doing this today.

Second, you can look back and know that every day, you put something useful into your head. Take solace in the fact that you spent time developing your subconscious. You did something. You took action. You completed a rep—and most likely days, weeks, and years, of those reps. This is another small Inch Block moving you and your Mindset into the person and athlete you want to become. This successful action further builds confidence.

Third, if nothing else, you should have learned something. If you have half a brain, you will select something worthwhile and useful. And smarter people are harder to kill. Reading more worthwhile books versus watching documentaries will help you improve. At some point in your career, young athleticism will deteriorate. You'll need your accumulated wisdom to compensate. And yet the task will remain the same: Win. At various stages, you'll need different tools and capabilities. Get smarter now. It's at least a necessity and a competitive advantage. Getting smarter in your craft will build confidence.

Fourth, this set of actions reinforces and solidifies the concept of "process." You and anyone can develop a systematic process to improve in an area. With a finite number of minutes in a day, you can spend a fraction of those minutes in a specific, strategic, and deliberate way. You will have taught yourself and lived through this process, and you'll believe it's repeatable. Simply reapply it in your next chosen endeavor.

CHAPTER 15

MINDSET - CONFIDENCE AND TOUGHNESS

This one is very simple. Not easy. But very, very simple. Confidence comes from reps. Toughness comes from reps. That's it. Your job is to get more reps than the other guy, quicker than the other guy, and harder reps than the other guy. Now. This section is how we move forward.

Programming Yourself

We already discussed brainwashing yourself. Have you scheduled that into your day? There was a process for this activity. It's critical, especially early on in your career. Remember, you're doing this now so you know you can conduct the necessary tasks. Once you know you can, then you switch your Mindset to "You must do this." But when?

Morning Routine

Before we progress further with the different topics, we need to stop and introduce two basics for your Inches Process. First is the morning routine. Structure and habits are requirements for success and winning. They're as important as breathing if you equate winning with that level of dedication. Set your day up for success at once. I guarantee you that it's critical to your improvement.

Remember, above I said, "Confidence comes from reps." The morning is when we start. Recall there are six Inch Blocks of improvement in this book (Mindset, Knowledge, Teammates, Training, Nutrition, and Recovery). In each section, you learn where to add new tasks and habits to your day. For some people, their habits are suited better for the morning, and others are better for the evening. Still others could be during the day. Different habits and tasks may occur daily, while other habits only occur weekly, monthly, and quarterly. All are important. You will see that you will become the sum of your habits, right or wrong. Like it or not. It's coming for you regardless of your belief in that fact. If you don't add any new habits to your morning, then guess what? That is your habit. Progress slows down, and you're not improving in the morning. Remember, you are the sum of your habits.

Here are the targets. Add one before you add two. You can't improve a habit until you have the habit:

- Get up at the same time every day. Fluctuate as little as possible on the weekends. Why? Consistency makes it easier on your internal body clock. If you fly across the country and change the time zone, it creates jet lag. Your body doesn't like that. It's inefficient. So don't do it to yourself unless it's unavoidable. Later when you're a pro, you can evolve to Tim Grover's approach to different rising times to prepare yourself for the constant jet lag from pro travel.
- Set as many alarms as you need to get up at the necessary time. Move the alarms away from your bed so you must get up.
- Knock out your bathroom basics.
- Take in a glass of water to jump-start your metabolism. Take in any necessary supplements.

- Make your bed and straighten your living area at once. Discipline is a Core Value. Become Disciplined throughout the day and your endeavors. It will shape your identity. Then when the time comes, you'll have the confidence to know you'll crush the task because of your consistent Discipline.
- Do something physical at once. It activates your nervous system and continues to jump-start your metabolism. I usually walk the dogs. We walk between one to three miles. Sometimes I wear a weighted ruck (large backpack with weight between forty and seventy pounds.) Other times I don't use the ruck at all. We walk in every version of weather: seventy-five degrees and 90 percent humidity, heavy rain, zero degrees and windy, and nice days too. I walk through the neighborhoods or travel to a local park. But I move daily. (Again, I'm not perfect. No one is. But this sets the tone for me.) Are you in your room instead? Great. Then do eight to fifteen minutes of a circuit: Fifteen push-ups, thirty flutter kicks, and a thirty-second plank hold. Just move.
  - While I'm walking, I can listen to podcasts or hype videos for brainwashing, or I can pick a topic to mull over in my head. Or I can let my mind go and declutter. Sometimes it's just fun country music. Other times, it's aggressive music to get my head right for a heavy lifting session. Or I could calm down and talk with Jesus and pray.
- Mindset Reps. The next few bullet points are a brief outline of what to do in the morning for managing your day. I will lay out a structured approach for what to do in the Process section of the book. I will bring everything together so you will have a systematic process for each Inch Block. The following is for you to look over and get a sense of what we will be doing eventually. That's it.
  - Write down one thing you're grateful for. Six months ago, you would've killed to be at this point. Don't forget that.
  - What are your main obstacles you face today?
  - Look at your calendar so you know the time constraints.

- ◦ Meditate for five minutes.
- ◦ Take an ice bath or cold shower for five minutes.
- ◦ What is your mantra for today? This word or phrase will guide your approach to the day's challenges.
- Eat like a winner. Don't botch this step. You'll need a plan here to execute. We'll discuss this further in the Nutrition section.
- If you drive somewhere next, then add in more Brainwashing. You don't have to do this every time. But if you never do, then your score is zero. So, when you are debating on doing the required work to improve, then revisit your "Whys" for competing.

At this point, your morning is well on its way. You've already done a ton. And it will show. Take the old Army approach: "We accomplish more before 6:00 a.m. than you do all day." It's why Jocko Willink is up at 4:30 a.m. Eric Thomas is up at 3:00 a.m. The old motivational speaker Jim Rohn was once asked why he was always up so early. He responded, "If you were going where I am and had to do what I have to do, then you'd be up early too."

If this were your morning routine, would you develop confidence? Of course you would. You're now a doer. You get hard, meaningful things done. You are training your subconscious as well. You are finding tasks and obstacles. You're on the attack. You're moving forward! That's the point. Get better. Beat your opponent. Beat yesterday's version of you. Get up and win.

Evening Routine

Makes sense, right? How you begin and end your days makes an impact. Let's be great and finish strong. See it all the way through. Sisu is a Core Value. Never quit. That also means finishing the tasks to completion. You know when it's complete. Be strong and get it right.

- Mindset Reps: Journal
  - How did you perform with the six main Inch Blocks? What went well? What did you learn?
  - Your selected mantra was your overarching guiding phrase for the day. How well did you stay true to it?
  - Why are you grateful?
  - What's big for tomorrow?
  - Pray or meditate.
- Thirty to sixty minutes to go: Stop with the phone. Stop with the TV. Stop with the computer. Give your mind a break. Now remember, this is best. I get it that with limited time, sometimes you'll work right to the end and head to bed. I'm not naïve either. You could be with your spouse or boyfriend/girlfriend, or even your bad mistake "hookups." That happens too. But ideally, the stimulus stops now, and your mind can make the transition to resting.
- Keep your environment as cold as possible. Your brain loves the cold. Your body, not so much. So use whatever blankets you like.
- Get rid of the light in the room so your eyes don't send images to your brain.
- Play background white noise. You can run a fan for the noise or download an app on your phone that plays the sound of waves, rain, or the wind.
- Don't drink fluids late at night. You want to sleep. You don't want to be up using the bathroom all night. Discipline matters. Consume your fluids earlier in the day.
- If you're a big guy, you may need a CPAP to maximize oxygen intake.
- If you want a quality mattress, then go to www.cravemattress.com. It's great.
- Get a Chillow Cooling Pillow (on Amazon). It's a cold pillow that's great to sleep on.

- Have your room in order so you aren't living in chaos.
- Other than the alarm, turn your phone off. (It's worth repeating this habit to yourself.)
- I like an extra pillow between my legs for when I sleep on my side. It helps with my spine alignment and takes pressure off my lower back.

More reps = More confidence. Now you're living your Mindset. You're training it again. You are on your path, and movement gets you there. The point is to move forward. And now you are. Good.

Toughness

Becoming tougher is simply a result of handling tougher reps. Being tough is the opposite of being a coward. Both the tough guy and coward experience fear. The difference is that the tough guy never backs down from fear. He is consistently in uncomfortable situations. He systematically toughens himself up by handling harder and harder challenges. That's it. He doesn't win every battle. And he doesn't fight every battle either. But when he must battle, he's all in or not at all. He won't ever back down then. This must be you too. And you get there by doing harder tasks, harder reps.

Flipping the Switch.

Sport needs conflict. No one watches you play basketball against yourself. Sport at any level is intense. It's also relative intensity. The seven-year-olds are trying hard to get the soccer ball to themselves, travel the length of the field with it, and score. The winner is going full out. The pro is going full out as well. However, the game of soccer is obviously different at the two levels. It doesn't even appear to be the same sport. But it is. And winning requires intensity at the highest level.

The highest levels of intensity aren't sustainable throughout the day. Sometimes they're not sustainable throughout a single game. At times, you must "flip the switch" as one of our coaches, Dustin Burford, would say. Tim Grover calls it "being in the zone." At that moment, focus is at its peak. You home in on one target at a time, and you pursue it until you have it or it's over. I saw this old clip of Ed Reed. Reed is a Hall of Famer for the Baltimore Ravens. The clip had him on the punt team against the Indianapolis Colts. Reed is rushing the punter, and the blocker holds Reed back by snagging his face mask. That's a penalty, and the ref missed it. Reed is irate, screaming at the ref. Nothing happens in the split-second Reed is screaming. Well, Reed finds the guy downfield that face-masked him. Reed takes off like Michael Johnson running the hundred-meter in the Olympics. He lowers his shoulder and head at the Colt and launches the Colt, who crumbles to the field. Done. Reed "flipped the switch" in the moment and decided to make an impact on that play. He did.

The Reed example is for one play. You can flip the switch as you enter onto the field. You make a conscious decision to put all thoughts out of your head. Your only concern is your job on each play. Execute. Execute violently, Relentlessly. That's flipping the switch.

You can flip the switch when you rise in the morning too. It's game day. You go about your business all day long. As the game approaches, your focus increases. You have a set playlist that gets your mind right. You dress differently. You eliminate calls and distractions. It's game day! Gotta go!

The key part for flipping the switch is the approach that in this moment, game, or day, you decide that you will put out all efforts to carry out your objective. It's "win or die trying." Pain and consequences have no meaning. It's only the task required to win. The end. It takes that level of commitment.

When I would have a heavy back squat in the gym that day, the entire session was different. Often, the thought would start creeping into my head the night before. The morning of would be different too. My head would be down during warm up and between sets so I could look at the floor. I didn't want to engage with others and get distracted. There were only four or five songs I'd listen to as the top sets approached. Then, for each set when it was time to go through my routine and squat, the only word I'd utter was "Up!" I knew that that one of two things would occur: Either I would stand up successfully with the bar on my back myself, or I would stand up with the help of spotters. But there was no way the bar was going down and staying down. For me, it was the belief that I'd stand up for myself no matter what. All I had to do was keep pushing up before I passed out from lack of oxygen. Perfect. Problem solved! And once the set was over, I'd calm down a little and prepare for the next set.

Resolve

Occasionally there is employee turnover at my gym. It's not often, but it does happen. Years ago, two ladies coached for me. They started their own nutrition business out of my gym as well. Then one day, they decided to quit and leave. Their nutrition business moved five miles away along with them. They hoped to coach for a local competitor or potentially open their own gym to compete with mine. I was supremely stupid for not requiring a noncompete agreement with them at first. It was an amateur mistake. In this instance, it cost me very little because they could never compete with our product or service. But it had the potential to really hurt me.

Well, that mistake was one and done. I added noncompete agreements that even our interns must sign. The terms of the agreement are clear in the document. In addition, I supply a verbal warning as well. It typically sounds like this: "You and I both now understand the non compete. But also, know this: that if you try to steal from me, then you and I are going to fight. Straight up. And you might win. But you will hurt and suffer in the process. I do not care about the legal ramifications. Steal from me, and I will hurt you."

At that point, the die is cast, and I am past the point of no return. I have resolve. I've decided. This is the line in the sand. Cross it, and I flip a switch. I unlock a preset path. There will be moments or days when this will be necessary for you as well. Resolve that on this play, no one gets by you. Resolve that this game, there are no plays off. Resolve that today is the day that you get more done than anyone else. Resolve that this season, you are the best tackler on the team, that your passes are better than all others, that you watch more film than your teammates, that you stand for something huge! Your resolve becomes your identity. When that moment arises, you must execute. Move forward aggressively.

Headbutt First

In different situations, you will have to fight. It usually arises from bullying. A teammate. An opponent. Someone. The point isn't that you need to look for fights. It's also not that you should engage in fighting easily either. It's very rare that fighting is the way to go. However, you may have to let someone, or a group of people, know that they can't bully you any longer. Your message must be clear: Messing with you means severe pain.

In this instance, headbutt them first. And if it's against a group, go at the biggest guy first. If it really is go time, then go and go all out. Go hard. And don't let up until it is clearly over. In the literal sense, yes, headbutt them square in the nose and it could be over instantly. But beat his ass anyway just to make sure. It's your best chance.

In the metaphoric sense, it won't require a physical altercation or fight. If you're a defender in soccer, then maybe no opponents advance the ball into your territory. Otherwise, you will provide so much pressure that he turns the ball over repeatedly. This is more likely the "fight" you're in. And you fight just as hard as if you were in a back-alley brawl. You just do so on the field.

Laura Phelps is the best pound-for-pound powerlifter of all time. She was a competitive lifter in the 90s and into the early 2000s throughout the United States. The sport of powerlifting is composed of three lifts for maximum weight: the back squat, the bench press, and the deadlift. The lifter's total is the sum of the three lifts. For context, Phelps's best total was more than eleven times her body weight. Let that sink in for a second. There was one meet where she and the other main opponent were neck and neck right up to the end. And for the life of me, I can't recall who won. But it was very close, within 5–10 kg (11–22 lb.), and it could've been her opponent. That is not the point. The point is that Phelps's opponent taunted her afterward.

Then about nine months went by, and there was another huge meet in the US with good prize money for the winner. The meet always starts with the back squat. Each lifter in a heat warms up, and then everyone in the heat goes through their first attempts. Then each lifter in the heat has a second attempt, and finally the third and final attempt. The first heat had Phelps's main opponent (the same one that beat her nine months prior). When the heat finished, Phelps's opponent had set a new all-time world record in the back squat. Amazing, right? It truly was. She came to play.

But Phelps was in the next heat. Phelps's opening weight, her first attempt, was well over the brand-new world record. It was a new record and Phelps still had two lifts left! Her next two attempts continued to climb and further smash the records. And then she did the same thing in the bench press and finally the deadlift. It wasn't even close.

Going into the meet in her opponent's mind, she was either a little bit ahead of Phelps or a little bit behind her. Either way, she was close. She had what you don't ever want to give an opponent: hope. Hope is powerful, and you must not give your opponent any. You must crush it in your opponent when possible. However, over that next training period, Phelps took her training to an unprecedented level and distanced herself fully. She beat her opponent so badly that she never competed again. Done. Quit. Over. No Sisu in her. This isn't a literal example of headbutting someone and fighting. But it was a fight, nonetheless. And Phelps went at her and crushed her so badly, she didn't get back up. That's the point. Phelps continued on to more titles and successes. She now owns and runs her own gym in the Cincinnati area. If you can find her, she is a true master of her craft and can get you stronger. Check her out.

In both circumstances, a literal fight and a fight on the field or court, do the same thing. Strike hard with all you have. And keep going until you cross the finish line, win the game, and come out on top.

Arrive Earlier. Leave later.

Most say work smarter, not harder. Wrong. Work smarter *and* harder. Increase efficiency? You bet your ass you need to do that. Yes, work smarter. Add that to an unbeatable work ethic, and then you have a shot. Eric Thomas always talks about being up at 3:00 a.m. to start his day to outwork his competitors. If you go on his social media, you'll see his posts and live videos occur then too. He's no liar. He works his butt off. If you add that work ethic with advances in technology, habits, and new methods, that's unbeatable. And I'm not saying Thomas doesn't do that. I'm saying always do both. Kaizen means being 1 percent better in all aspects. That means your work ethic too.

James Clear highlights perfecting your environment for improved performance. The big driver in this endeavor is eliminating distractions. All right then. Be on the court or field or in the weight room first. No one is there. No distractions. Perfect. Now get work done.

Watch the ESPN documentary about Tom Brady, *The Man in The Arena*. There's a segment where Brady and his main core of teammates taunt each other about "getting the edge." Brady would ask, "How many hours of film did you get in today? Oh, only two hours? I'll get two and a half hours." Or "How many hours of treatment? Oh, forty-five minutes? Great. I'll get sixty minutes." He'd always end with "looking like I'm getting the edge on you."

So, how do you know when to stop working? How do you find a balance? The reality is that you'll be out of balance for a good long while. How long? Until you stop competing. So, get that misconception out of your head. There is no balance for greatness. On the other side, you can't watch film for twenty-four hours each day. You have other things to do, like eat, sleep, lift, and practice. These basic habits will guide you:

- Go past a level of discomfort. Always. If the task requires sixty minutes of work, then schedule an extra thirty minutes just in case.
- If you must complete something, then you already know the answer. Get it done. Now. And do it right the first time.
- Set up sustainable habits. Sustainability is a requirement, not a suggestion. Schedule it. You need thirty minutes of treatment a day? Then get in and get it done. Don't schedule a three-hour massage once every two weeks. Get tiny amounts done daily. The same is true with film study. Schedule a sustainable amount of time daily.
- Arrive early and stay late. There is a chapter in James Kerr's book, *Legacy*. It simply says, "Champions do more." It's true. Similarly, one of Urban Meyer's mantras in his book, *Above the Line*, is "Everything you do + 2." Meaning, always do two more reps in all assignments. All of them.

A Disproportionate Response

Coaches will evaluate you. There will be times when your boss or coach or someone is really trying to stick it to you. It may be a bullying experience. It could be someone talking crap to you on the court. Here's a true and potentially painful reality: It will often be your good friends communicating tremendous doubt toward you and your abilities. Your "friends" (who may need to go) will tell you that your goals are impossible, that you can't do something. People will try to treat you like garbage all the time if you let them. Others' insecurities will come shining through. They could disrespect you. It's an unfortunate reality.

Now it's time for a disproportionate response. It's time to show them and prove them wrong. It's time to take on Michael Jordan's most common phrase in *The Last Dance*: "I took that personal." Whoever the idiot is who's calling out to you and calling your family name needs to understand that you will do what you say you will do. You follow through and kick your opponent's butt, so he cracks and gives up. You take his spirit and will. David Goggins calls it "taking souls" in his book, *Can't Hurt Me*. And Goggins is right! Do it. Hammer on a project so much that you're done well ahead of others. Someone says you're too slow to compete. Then get strong and fast as possible. You're too dumb to understand the playbook? Master it so well you can teach it to the coach. You can't break a tackle? Buy a harness and chain and attach it to your car to pull it. Build your reputation so you are known to be reliable. You want to be known as the guy who delivers. You are the one who gets the results. At the higher levels in sports, only results matter.

What's the process? Pick any example. Take the playbook example above as the challenge. Ask the person accusing you of not knowing it to quantify what will prove to him that you are a master of the playbook. You're a running back, and he says you're too dumb to know the plays. But if you know all your assignments, then you would qualify as an "expert" in his eyes. Since the criteria have been set, you do this, in this order:

- Memorize your assignments fully as the running back.
- Memorize the assignments of all the offensive lineman fully because if they are doing their job right or wrong, it will affect you.
- Memorize the assignments of the receivers in the same fashion.
- Then know the assignments for different defensive fronts and changes at the line of scrimmage.
- Set a date and time.

- Let that person know what a real master of the playbook looks like.

Do you get it now? It's the same approach as everything else we are doing here. Find the target. Outwork everyone, so it's noticeable and embarrassing to the competition. Over-execute and win. Repeat. Relentlessly

Need another example? You fumbled at football practice and the coach got on you because fumbles equal losses in games. And he should have. It's true. Turnovers = Losses = Players Getting Demoted = Coaches Losing Jobs = Money Lost for Everyone. What's your response? If I were coaching you, I'd run you through every ball-handling drill, so you are unstoppable. Then I'd make your grip and arm strength Arnold Schwarzenegger-strong. Your target to prove the point will be to set the conference record for the number of carries without a fumble. "Oh, you're worried because I made a mistake. Got it. How about I smash a record? Now I'm known for being the most reliable athlete on the field. Go ahead and draft me because I'm the best. Next?"

Seek Pain and Discomfort.

Conflict occurs often, sometimes daily. Embrace it and run to it. Conflict managed well improves relationships and builds confidence. Conflicted managed poorly or avoided destroys relationships and ruins confidence. Stop and think about this. It's a truism or equation that works. Believe me. Or don't believe me; that's fine. I'll show you here in a second that it's true nonetheless.

Let's start in the gym. Back squat. When you lift, it's you versus you and you versus the bar. It's you versus the doubts, fears, and issues. It's you versus injury. It's you versus persevering, attacking, and getting stronger, and it's you versus giving up, shying away, and getting weaker. When does this occur? At first, it's fearful to get into the gym at all.

Simply going will improve performance naturally. Then increased confidence is the natural byproduct. Confidence comes from reps.

Eventually, going to the gym isn't a big deal. Why? Because it's not! But now it's squat day (best day of the week!), and you are instructed to work up to a one-rep max. In this example, your current max is 315 lb. The target becomes 320 lb. if everything looks and feels decent that day. If you come in with the flu or are crushed from school/work and lack of sleep, then today is not the day to evaluate a max, typically. Assuming you're good to go, then go!

You work your way up the lifting ladder. 295 lb. or 305 lb. looked good. So the coach tells you to put on 325 lb. It's your next lift, and you go through your routine again. (Nothing changes. Routine is critical.) There are two potential outcomes: You hit 325 lb. and feel good. You miss 325 lb. and feel not so good. There is conflict there. How it's managed decides everything. I love Tim Knight's equation: E + R = O. Event + Response = Outcome. The Event is *not* the Outcome. Only you can decide the Outcome. Follow along here with this scenario and decide how you will manage it in the future:

Scenario 1: You make the lift.

Naturally, you'll feel good because you progressed. Forward motion and improvement are the goals. How did the lift look? On a "max effort lift," the weaknesses in the body and mind will become clear. Even if you make it, you'll pick up clues on what is lagging. Or hopefully your coach or spotters pick up on the clues. For example, if your knees cave in while you make the lift, it shows your glutes are the lagging muscle group. For the foreseeable future you must strengthen all parts of your butt muscles to advance. Hunt for weaknesses. Write them down. Devise a solution and course of action. Then continue to execute and improve.

Scenario 2: You miss the lift.

Why? And why again? And why again? What changed? It could be any of the following factors:

- Were you "in your head" and afraid of the lift? Did you doubt yourself?
- Were you distracted and not focused?
- When it got hard and started to move slowly, did you give up? I've seen people stop the lift while the bar is still moving forward in the right direction.
- Then there is the physical side: knees cave in? Chest and core collapse? Get too far forward and out of position? Drop too low in the bottom? Take too long in the lift and stop due to fatigue? Black out during the lift?
- Now, how did you respond? I'd be mad as hell. If I missed the lift because of a mental mistake, then I'd be supremely angry. Then I'd have to watch the video to see what happened. (Record your PR attempts in all lifts to assess flaws. Always.) At this point, you must identify the flaws, devise a plan to improve them, and execute.

In both scenarios, you'll notice that the final thing to do is the same. You must find what went well and what did not. It's not more complicated and involved than that. But it must occur. The information is the most valuable part of the lift! Why? Because you need to know what the limiting factors are. I'm sure you've heard that a chain is only as strong as its weakest link. It's true. You must find what part is weak in your lift. If you don't, you cannot improve. And that is unacceptable. Win or lose. You must find the next target. There is another phrase, "You either win or you learn." This phrase comes up a little short and is incorrect. The winning only occurs *if* you learn because without the learning, you cannot win again. If you do not learn in both scenarios, then you take a loss. Why? Because the only play that means anything, the only lift that matters, the only opportunity that matters is the next one.

CHAPTER 16

MINDSET - PRESSURE

W hat is it? It's most likely this: An important deadline in your sport or at work or tasks is quickly approaching. You must do something. The results are important to you because you want something. Typically, it's that you want to feel a certain way. Add the fact that the task is hard and challenging. You probably perceive that your reputation and therefore your ego is on display. You want to look a certain way. You want to win. You want to be strong, not weak. You want to be liked and respected, not loathed and hated. You want fame and money, not obscurity and poverty.

Ultimately pressure (or fear) just tells you that what is about to occur is important to you for any number of reasons. That's it.

Here is how Mark Divine describes it in *The Way of The Seal*. The future has a VUCA structure:

V: Variable. The event. For the context of this book, let's choose to look at practice or a game. Yes. The plays and outcomes have a multitude of variables.

U: Uncertain. This is true. We don't know exactly what the variables will be. We can guess. And we can make solid, educated guesses. But it is still uncertain.

C: Complex. Definitely. Playing in the peewee league for soccer just means everyone swarms to the ball like bees to honey. In football, it's run left, run right, run up the middle, and one pass per game. In the pros, soccer players bend the path of the ball from the corner kick to someone lunging headfirst into the pass to send it into a net past a series of defenders and a diving goalie. In football, five different checkdowns occur on offense and defense before the ball is snapped. Then another dozen options unfold as elite players simply try to move a ball one yard.

A: Ambiguous. Absolutely. Each play, each team, each time you face the same team, each venue, each player, each version of the weather is unknown. Anything can happen.

Look at it from Dane Jensen's perspective in his book, *Power of Pressure*. For him it's an equation:

Pressure = Importance × Uncertainty × Volume

You'll see recurring themes here. The event is important to you. No one knows exactly how it will unfold. And there is a lot going on leading up to the event and during the event itself. What's more, the event is rarely a one-time deal. Even the Olympics occur every four years. You must still perform in high school, college, and national-level events multiple times for your shot at the Olympics.

There is pressure over the long-term and more intense pressure in the short-term. In the weight room, you might squat twice per week, usually at lower weights for speed and higher reps. There is physical and mental pressure to squat well each week to build strength and power. Occasionally, you'll also squat at your heaviest ever. Long-term, there is some pressure, and there is intense pressure in the short-term. You physically feel the pressure when you are under the bar at heavier and heavier loads.

There is pressure to play well in high school if you want a chance to play in college. In college you're with the top 7 percent (depending on the sport) and you must play well in practice just to make it to the game field. Then you need to be the best on your team (unless you're Ohio

State and Alabama) to get drafted or invited to make an NFL roster. During camp, 53 of 80 make it onto the team. You see my point? Each level of success requires more and coincides with more pressure.

Who doesn't know that? Right. How do you handle it? What's the process? Those are the meaningful questions.

Short Term: Game, Moment

The main step in everything is preparation. This statement applies to the short and long terms. It's obvious. But we will state the obvious as well. "It's not the will to win. It's the will to prepare." – Bobby Knight. Prepare like a driven athlete as if your life depends on it, and you'll be fine. Why? Because that level or prep requires so much work that you must feel confident. And the feeling of pressure will be almost minimal. You'll simply execute.

Focus

Your ability to direct your focus will account for most of your results. James Kerr's *Legacy* summarizes it as RedHead (tight, inhibited results-oriented, anxious, aggressive overcompensating, desperate) versus Blue Head (loose, expressive, in the moment, calm, clear, accurate, on task). Be a Blue Head. But how?

Blue Head Process

1. Recognize the situation (pre-game, warm-ups, in between plays, etc.).

2. Recognize how you feel and how you typically feel: heart rate, breathing, sweating, anxiety—what?

(Note: These two answers you should know by now. I'm sure you've played before. So, write down how you feel in different scenarios.)

3. Learn what you need to do in these situations. What you do will change how you feel. Not fully. But it will give you a better shot.

4. Breath. Five deep breaths. Ten if possible. Calm your body.

5. Anchor yourself. Look at something outside the element. Look at a tattoo you have, look at a point in the stands, look at a flag. Me? I make the sign of the cross with my thumb on the palm of my hand.

6. Assess the next step. Maybe it's just warm-ups. Most likely, it is the next play or series of plays. You must know your job. Like an expert. "Just do your job," screams Bill Belichick on most plays in practice and in the game. What is the one thing you can do very well right now that will make an impact? What would a college athlete do, a pro, the one at the Statue level?

7. Know. Know that you put in a ton of work and had great successes leading to this point. You can do it. You have done it in the past. You can do it again. Focus on your mantra and go!

8. Mantra. What is your word(s) for the day or game? You should be reciting your mantra in your morning ritual as you do five minutes of meditating. As my son Jack was prepping for games in his second season at Ball State, his mantra became F&P. "Fast and physical." It's a must for linebackers and most on the field.

9. When it's time to go, it's either full speed and all out, or it's nothing. You choose a path for that moment. It's all in. No one did anything great in life or in a moment in a game going half speed or three-quarters speed. Go hard or don't go at all. In fact, just go home if you go in soft.

10. Learn. Do this on each play, after each practice or game. Write down the lessons in your evening journal.

11. Evolve and adjust. Daily. Apply what you learned. You're not fast enough? Adjust your training. You're slow to react on a play? More hours of film study alone and with a teammate. Struggle to calm down? Practice meditating in the morning and put yourself in stressful situations in your life.

I listed what to do in the moment. Practice it until you never need to. Also, in these peak moments, get rid of all the crap around that isn't necessary. Distractions hurt focus. Get rid of them. Turn off your phone. Get your home life scheduled and taken care of. Harder the task means less time for crap.

Basic example: You're trying to make the freshman basketball team. Get your homework done, room and laundry clean, and get your food packed. Turn off your phone. Practice and prepare. Go give them hell.

Extreme example: You're LeBron James trying to win your first NBA title. Hire someone to take care of all home life, rides, food, media, tickets—anything, and everything. Turn off your phone. Practice and prepare. Go give them hell.

Lastly, look back at the example of my grandfather, Alton Beebe. When he compared his ability to make a living for his family to surviving World War II, it was no comparison. He could always make more money and provide for his family. On the other end of the spectrum, he survived almost getting his face shot off in the war. And he survived the war in Europe and North Africa. Making the team or winning the game is huge and amazing. But it is not life and death. And it is not a world-changing life or a World War. Perspective. Recognize the moment for what it is. Be "all in" with each moment. Simply understand the difference in the importance in your life.

Long Term

Prepare and prepare some more. Work harder. Work smarter. Move forward!

Look back at your Levels of "Why." The clearer and harsher the "Why," the easier it is to persevere. Revisit that. Look deep inside. Find yourself all over again. This will help sustain you. But it will not carry you every day. It won't. Won't! Find new "Whys". Find more "Whys." Renew them daily. Find other simple motivations. Find other simple wins. And even when you run out here, Discipline is a Core Value! Keep moving forward. Prepare when you want to—and also when you don't want to any longer.

Revisit the piece on change. Change is a constant. It's a VUCA life. It's a VUCA sport. Evolve or die. New Level = New Challenges. Extreme Level = Extreme Challenges.

Personal Example. In early 2013, I opened my gym. It grew to twenty to thirty members in the first month. I coached all the sessions, handled all the chores of the gym, and handled all the management jobs of the gym. Hard, right? As of late 2022, we have about two hundred adult and student athletes at any point in time. We have a staff of twelve CrossFit coaches, outsourced admins, and professionals, and as of this writing, I'm revamping the sport performance aspect because my head coach just quit. We offer the most events of any gym in the Midwest. Our gym raises the most money of any gym for charity in Indiana. We added nutrition coaching, mindset training, and more. I rarely coach at all now. Which is harder? Does it even matter which is harder? I know in five years we will continue to evolve, or the business will die. You must do the same. Ultimately, I keep advancing. I look for larger and more important problems to solve in the long term and short term. It's fun for me.

If you must chop wood all day, take breaks to sharpen your ax. Make it easier. In this exact moment, September 14, 2022 at 11:36 a.m., I am in Brown County State Park writing at a picnic table in the woods. I take a "corporate retreat" four times a year to reassess things in the business. I take a step back and look around and assess things. I'm also using this time to write feverishly. Throughout the year, I travel with my family to enjoy our life. As much as possible, I hike on Wednesday mornings in the woods to calm down. The point? Everyone must rest and recover. Working like a maniac is not sustainable in the long term. People break. If not break, they at least don't perform optimally if they never rest and recover. Plan it out. Make it happen. The nervous system can only take so much. Rest and sleep are the only ways to bring it back.

Pain doesn't show up for no reason. Pain is inevitable. Suffering is not. Examine what the pain is trying to teach you. Maybe the pain is terrible, maybe it's great. 1 James: "Be grateful for the suffering, for it causes perseverance." Example: You're in football practice, and on a play, you get "blown up" and pancaked on defense. It hurts. It's humiliating (if you care what others think). And the coach calls you out. Coach questions your manhood and your ability to play. You just took an L, right? Maybe. Maybe not.

Maybe you believe the coach. Your confidence goes down. It seeps into your psyche. You don't prepare as much because you believe him. Next practice, you're down, so you're playing slowly. As a result, you're out of position. You make another mistake and you do it again. You couldn't handle the adversity, which means you won't be able to handle the next level of adversity. Coach recognizes this. So down the depth chart you go.

Maybe not. "I'll show you coach!" you say to yourself. "Yeah, I made a mistake on this play. I was playing slow because I wasn't fully cognizant of the plays you changed. Okay. I accept that. Now, watch this!" Again, all to yourself. That night, two extra hours of film study. Tomorrow, the same thing with others in the surrounding positions to know each other better. Write about it in your journal at night. More notes every night thereafter. Up early to clear my head, meditate, work on my mantra: "Smart and pain." Here is the thought process: I'm going to be the smartest one on the field, knowing all the ins and outs of the job. And I am going to cause pain for everything and everyone in my way. Is someone trying to block me? They'll feel enough pain that they move. Someone with the ball? They'll feel enough pain that they go down.

Coach not playing me? He'll feel enough pain from those around him that he'll put me in. There will be so much pain for the coach from bad results from not playing me and so much pleasure for him when he does play me because of all the great plays I will make that change must occur. Either get him fired for not playing the best player on the team or make him coach of the year for when he does play you.

CHAPTER 17

MINDSET - WAY OF INCHES

Time to work. This Block is critical. The most critical. In Gary Keller's award-winning book, *The ONE Thing*, this would be The ONE Thing. Why? Because it is! Your mind makes all your decisions. And your decisions dictate your actions. And your actions dictate your results. You are where you are because your Mindset put you there. The end.

Mindset SWOT Analysis. (Strengths, Weaknesses, Opportunities, and Threats)

- Strength:
    - List them all.
    - What are your top three?
    - What is your number one Strength (Competitive Advantage)?
- Weaknesses:
    - List them all.
    - What are your top three?
    - What is your number one Weakness (Weak Link)?
- Opportunities:
    - List them all.
    - What are your top three?

- ◦ What is your number one Opportunity (Target)?
- • Threats:
  - ◦ List them all.
  - ◦ What are your top three?
  - ◦ What is your number one Threat (Enemy)?

Be sure to prioritize and identify your Competitive Advantage and your Weak Link. You must advance in these areas to optimize your performance. What is your number one Target for this quarter? Write out your process goals and habits for the next quarter. Share with your Mindset accountability ally. Your ally is someone you talk to at least weekly, and he or she holds you accountable. Devise your carrot (rewards) and stick (punishments) for how you do each week. See if you can find a mentor as well. It will be a huge boost if you can find someone to help coach you on the side. I can't imagine a scenario where you work this diligently and don't advance. It's impossible. You'll continue to crush it.

Let's revisit the Assessment Test for Mindset:

<u>MINDSET</u>

How well do you and others know your "Why"?

- • 10 Points: You know it; your unit knows it; your team knows it; your coaches know it; your support team knows it. You review it daily.
- • 8 Points: Two groups mentioned above know it. You review it at least four times a week.
- • 6 Points: You and your immediate Teammates know it. You review it weekly.

- 4 Points: You know it and review it monthly.
- 2 Points: You know it and review it quarterly.

POINTS: _____

How well do you and others know your Core Values?

- 10 Points: You know it; your unit knows it; your team knows it; your coaches know it; your support team knows it. You review it weekly.
- 8 Points: Two groups mentioned above know it. You review it at least weekly.
- 6 Points: You and your immediate Teammates know it. You review it weekly.
- 4 Points: You know it and review it monthly.
- 2 Points: You know it and review it quarterly.

POINTS: _____

What is your level of Integrity?

- 10 Points: You give maximum effort (90 percent or more) daily.
- 8 Points: You give 80 percent effort daily.
- 3 Points: You give 60 percent effort daily.
- 0 Points: All else.

POINTS: _____

What is your level of Enjoyment? How well do you reflect on positives, have gratitude, act humble, help others, and ultimately enjoy your sport?

- 10 Points: Daily
- 8 Points. Weekly
- 6 Points. Monthly
- 4 Points. Quarterly
- 0 Points: All else.

POINTS: _____

Sisu

- 10 Points: You never quit, ever. You push through all reps, see tasks to completion and beyond.
- 8 Points: You mostly complete all tasks to the fullest.
- 5 Points: You occasionally complete tasks to the fullest.
- 0 Point: All else.

POINTS: _____

Discipline

- 10 Points: You consistently do what must be done, when it must be done, beyond the minimums.
- 8 Points: You mostly do what must be done when it must be done.
- 5 Points: You occasionally do what must be done when it must be done.
- 0 Points: All else.

POINTS: _____

Kaizen

- 10 Points: You have a process for improving and adhere to it without fail.
- 8 Points: You mostly have a process and adhere to it.
- 5 Points: You occasionally have a process and adhere to it.
- 0 Points: All else.

POINTS: _____

Mindset Mentor

- 10 Points: You have one and connect weekly.
- 8 Points: You have one and connect monthly.
- 5 Points: You have one and connect quarterly.
- 0 Points: All else.

POINTS: _____

How effectively are you working with a Mindset accountability ally (or allies)?

- 10 Points: You and your ally review your results weekly, enforce a "carrot/stick," and adjust.
- 7 Points: You and your ally review your results monthly and sometimes enforce "carrot/stick."
- 4 Points: You and your ally review your results quarterly.
- 0 Points: All else.

POINTS: _____

You know your number one Mindset Strength (Competitive Advantage):

- 10 points. Otherwise: 0 points.

POINTS: _____

You know your number one Mindset Weakness (Weak Link):

- 10 points. Otherwise: 0 points.

POINTS: _____

You know your number one Mindset Opportunity (Target):

- 10 points. Otherwise: 0 points.

POINTS: _____

You know your number one Mindset Threat (Enemy):

- 10 points. Otherwise: 0 points.

POINTS: _____

TOTAL POINTS: _____
OVERALL AVERAGE (TOTAL POINTS / 14) _____

What is your score? Now, where must you be at the end of your current career? So far, if you're in high school, the end of your current career is the end of your senior season. If you're in college, then it's the end of your college senior season. For pros, it's when you retire. Think about it.

Where must you be at the end of the current season or year?

Where must you be at the end of the next quarter, in ninety days?

End of next month?

End of this week?

Today?

Great. Now we have a score. We have crucial information now (your "Whys," your values, your allies, etc.).

Sustainability. Getting overwhelmed and bogged down is the quickest way to quitting anything. (Reread James Clear's *Atomic Habits*.) Make it easy. Make it obvious. Make it attractive. Make it satisfying. Those are Clear's four rules for sustaining a habit.

Get four large sticky notes, one for each SWOT component. List your Competitive Advantage, Weak Link, Target, and Opportunity. Write out the habit or action you must complete. Schedule it and execute. Then make a "tick mark" for each time you work on a habit. Twelve tick marks = Carrot. Two days missed in a row = Stick. Remember, your Mindset Block is the most critical. It governs all actions. Therefore, you must continue to shape and construct your Mindset daily.

Take me for an example—not that I'm anywhere near the best father, but I'm working on it. At forty-eight years old, some new fathers in my gym will ask me for some basic advice on how to be a decent father. My answer has been the same for twenty years: "If you give a shit every day, you'll be just fine. And if you don't, you won't." Think about that statement. The statement doesn't give any tasks or things to do. There are no habits listed. I simply summarize what your Mindset must be to perform well. "Give a shit." Why? Because if you do care at all, then you'll learn new things to do as a father. You'll care and love your child. You'll work to shape and mold your child. You'll try hard, if nothing else, and then you'll work and do what's necessary. And you'll do it daily.

How else can you improve your chances of executing your tasks? Post a picture of your sticky notes on your phone, screensaver with your tablet or laptop, on your refrigerator, next to your headboard.

10 Mindset Habits

If you have no idea what habits could improve your Mindset, here are ten ideas. You need not do any of them or you could do them all. Do not add a second habit until the first habit is engrained and firmly set in your identity. Remember sustainability. Do not overwhelm yourself and quit. The following are in roughly order of preference, but it depends on you. You must decide.

1. Add in cold therapy. Start by taking fifteen seconds of a pure cold shower at the end of your shower, daily. Over the course of a year, work your way up to five minutes of either a cold shower or time in an ice bath daily. Learn to be uncomfortable every day and handle it.

2. Delete six items or people you follow on social media that are toxic. Add in six items or people on social media that help you improve.

3. Read something that help you improve daily. Minimum of ten pages or thirty minutes.

4. Walk outside daily to start your day for twenty minutes, regardless of weather. Think about what you must execute today to be great.

5. Listen to something motivational daily while you walk outside.

6. Meditate and/or pray for five minutes every morning to set your Mindset on the path you must have that day.

7. Journal your thoughts at the end of each day. Write down daily affirmations of where you will be and what you must do.

8. Add pain, discomfort, and challenges to your life. Add small ones daily and one large one each quarter. Confidence comes from reps. Show yourself you can handle more than you could last quarter. You'll build your warrior mindset.

9. Have a mantra that guides you. Pick one that is meaningful for you. In my son Jack's second year at Ball State, we came up with "fast and physical." This was how we was to practice and play for every rep. It became his Mindset.

10. Devise a plan and process for game day situations. Then further decide on a process for what to do during critical parts of your games. Execute.

<u>Scan the following QR code</u> or visit: https://athlete-builder.com to access and download the assessment in this chapter and other resources (free nutrition resources and free workout programs).

CHAPTER 18

KNOWLEDGE - HERE'S THE DEAL . . . .

All six Inch Blocks are critical to your success. You'll need to have the right Mindset to perform at your highest level (Mindset). You must be extremely knowledgeable in all areas inside and outside your sport (Knowledge). You must optimize your interactions with professional and personal teammates (Teammates). Physically, you must have all the tools to perform at a high level (Training). Then you'll need to fuel (Nutrition) and rest and heal (Recovery) after each day.

Your Mindset ties it all together. Your knowledge across the six Blocks is what you must increasingly learn. Applying what you learn is the process for constant improvement. Kaizen.

Your mind's job is to observe everything. Assess everything. Decide an action. Then your mind must make you act. Your mind's job is to force action. *Action*. Move forward! (I'm screaming this in my head to my laptop as I write this.) Action. Move forward.

If you're undisciplined and lazy, walk to the mirror and scream, beg, plead, and cuss yourself out to move forward. Every page here is written to get you to move forward. Daily. Consistently. Intensely. Your mind governs all. Develop it. My job here is to ask all the questions that you must answer. Your answers guide your development. Your answers are needed to outline paths and next steps. Then your mind must decide to move you forward.

Here are some questions to illustrate the point. What aspects of your mindset hurt your and help you (Mindset)? What do you truly know or not know about yourself and your tendencies (Knowledge)? What do you need to learn about your position coach so you can execute fully what he wants you to do (Teammates)? What parts of your training are wasting your time (Training)? How do you fuel yourself optimally on a road game that is three time zones away (Nutrition)? How do you bounce back from back spasms quickly so you can play the next day (Recovery)?

Essentially, you're looking to take your abilities as an athlete to the highest level you can. Simply stated, you must become a master of your sport. This takes a lifetime, and it works if, and only if, you spend your time improving in your sport. You must acquire the knowledge to survive, then thrive, and then win at a high level. It only occurs from a Relentless approach to improving. Learning every bit of your sport is critical.

Here are some more examples to help you hit home what I'm talking about. *Temet nosce.* Know thyself. Right out of James Kerr's *Legacy*:

Know thyself. Often attributed to Socrates, the phrase is even older, inscribed in the Inner Chamber of Luxor Temple, in Upper Egypt. "Man, know thyself," the hieroglyphs say, "and thou shalt know the gods."

Right out of Robert Greene's *Mastery*:

Da Vinci: "One can have no greater or smaller mastery than to master yourself."

Painful example: My junior year at St. Ignatius High School, I was working on my future career path in college. When I slowed everything down and stopped to think about it, I wanted to work in business in some fashion. I had no concrete idea, but I was leaning toward finance and life in the stock markets. My strongest areas in school were math and science. Consequently, several of my teachers strongly encouraged me to enter the engineering fields. It made sense. My parents thought so too. We visited the University of Michigan for engineering to learn more. I thought it seemed all right, like the "right thing to do." I let myself get swept up in the idea. So I applied to Michigan, Purdue, and Cincinnati and was accepted to all three for engineering. I didn't even apply to universities for business. Ultimately, I went to Purdue for engineering. . . and quickly hated engineering. Purdue was great. I simply hated the components of engineering. All of them. My third semester proved it too. I got a B in a required history course, a C in my third level of calculus, and Ds and Fs in my engineering courses. I was out. Purdue "invited me not to return." What major did I transfer into? Of course: business. It's where I wanted to be all along. Unfortunately, I had the pain of time lost and money wasted with out-of-state tuition. Both were very real to me as I covered most all my expenses after my first year. I either didn't know myself or lied to myself (which was much worse) and learned a hard lesson. You must learn how you work and respond in the world. Then you can adapt, act, and move forward. But you must learn.

Opportunity missed: Sixth grade was the first time I could play organized football. It was going to be a stretch too because I was rather big. For context, by eighth grade, I was 6′3″ and 190 lb. Well, there was a weight limit in junior high school, so this was my shot before high school. My parents and grandparents vehemently didn't want me to play. All I would hear was, "You'll get hurt. You'll get hurt. Don't do it." Well, when it came time to play, I was a fearful kid about it. Sure enough, I decided it "wasn't for me." Unfortunate in so many ways. Mainly because I let a fear decide for me (a brutal mistake). Not to mention that my high school team lost one game in four years and had three state titles and one national title. (Ugh!)

Fast forward to my first year in college. As a pledge in Kappa Alpha Order (a social fraternity) we had a full-contact football game against the active members. Turns out that when I got hit, I didn't die. It stung a little, but it was fun. Then when I would hit someone. . . well, then it really got fun. So, we put together a league of tackle games and had a fantastic time. I ended up loving it. I hadn't known that about myself, and I wish I did. Oh well. Move forward.

All right, you get the point about learning about yourself. Here is another point that is worth repeating, and I'll do so throughout the book. You already see that I am laying out steps to improve in the six areas. Again, do *not* start adding so many new things and habits that you get overwhelmed and quit. This is critical. Sustainability is what matters. Keep improving each week and month for a couple decades and see where you're at. Make small adjustments that last and occasionally you'll take a big leap forward with your daily habits. Stick to this approach. Adding ten new things one week won't work. Don't do it. Don't worry. I'll tie everything together so you can develop a systematic plan for improving. In these earlier chapters, simply note and write down the different ideas that could help you.

Knowledge

It's a bit awkward that Knowledge is one of the Inches components of success. Why? Well, you need increased Knowledge in the other five Inch Blocks. But you also need Knowledge in your sport. This is what we are about here: you playing your sport better! We will look at the Knowledge Block within your sport/craft first. Then we will explore the other five components briefly. We already discussed the Mindset side in prior chapters. The remaining four Blocks will be discussed later. Let's get to it.

In all things, assess where you are now. Decide to evolve to the next level. Execute. Reassess and move up again. Repeat Relentlessly. Recall I have four different levels of athlete:

• Pretender: This athlete doesn't really matter at all because he isn't going anywhere. He doesn't have "it" to be great. Now, it's fine to be at this level and work like a dog to advance. If you're at this level, get out of it immediately. Push hard. The main characteristic of a Pretender is that you don't have talent and you don't work your butt off.

• College: You're legit if you're at this level. You can and will play in college in some capacity.

• Pro: The percentage that get here are so small. . . . Wow. You're one of the few on the planet.

• Statue: Yup. You're at that immortal level. The future will remember you.

Recall the scoring metrics from the Assessment Test for how well you know your position. Let's assume you play tight end in football. Out of ten points:

• 5 Points: You know your position backward and forward. You know and execute all your routes. You know your blocking schemes. You know how to position your body and execute in all phases of the game. You know the different stances in footwork. You can position your body to catch the ball and take a hit. You know your job and can do it well.

• 6 Points: You know your job and the jobs of those nearest your position as well as you know your job. This would mean the other receivers and the linemen next to you (the tackles).

• 7 Points: At this level, you know the jobs of the entire offense. You won't know everything the QB does, but you are on the "same page" every time. This includes all the audibles and changes at the snap of each play. You also know the jobs of the receivers and running backs so if someone is "off" that play, then you can help get them in the right position.

- 8 Points: Here is where it's high-level smart. You know the defenses of all the teams in your conference because you see them the most often.
- 9 Points: Add in the defenses from your non-conference games and you're at a championship level.
- 10 Points: Only a handful are here. Ever. You have a file on any team you've faced. You know what the defensive coordinator and position coaches have tendencies to do. You are a master of exploiting their weaknesses.
- For context, Payton Manning, Tom Brady, and many others typically were at the facility studying film first of any on their team. They would get there at six in the morning to study and be last to leave. You must be obsessed to be the best. It must border on the religious. This is the level of Knowledge in your sport that you are working to over your career.

You must play fast, as fast as possible. This only occurs when you have mastery of your tasks. It's automatic at that point. You can play more on feel and instinct. You have supreme confidence because you know all the scenarios and permutations. If you don't feel you can play this way, it's understandable. It means you do not have mastery of your craft and work. . . yet. Add more reps, and you'll increase your mastery. Then and only then have you earned the right to have supreme confidence. Then you know it so well, you are a true expert.

What does "true expert" look like? Check out Malcolm Gladwell's *Outliers*, Greene's *Mastery*, and other references on mastery. There is not a set number of hours necessary for mastery. It takes what it takes. That said, a good standard is ten thousand hours. Some need more, others less. Ten years is also a good starting point. But get to cramming it in now! James Kerr's *Legacy* states that "Champions do more." It's true. So, get going here. Now.

Take this college example: One coordinator for Ball State was installing new plays on defense on Tuesday mornings. The team went over the plays that morning and went right to practice. I asked when the coach worked on the plays and devised them. Answer: 3:00–5:00 a.m. All right, then get to the facility in the 04:00 hour to get a jump on the plays before everyone else gets them at 5:00 a.m. If you need more time to learn, then you must schedule it. Getting up early is not hard. The hard part is going to bed early. Fix that problem, and you can get ahead. Get ahead, and you have a better shot to win.

For a high school example, Conner Duzan was an excellent soccer goalie for Plainfield High School in Indiana. The last sectional game was huge, and he knew he'd have to come up big. The game had the potential to come down to penalty kicks to end the game. That week, he went through his film study. He noted who typically performed the penalty kicks for the opposition. He then noted where each player typically kicked the ball. He wrote the kids' numbers and kick targets on his water bottle so he could check it between kicks. "It's not the will to win. It's the will to prepare." – Bobby Knight

Pro example: Dennis Rodman, Hall of Famer in the NBA, would simply sit and watch his teammates shoot. Then he'd watch film on others shooting. He was collecting data. He wanted to know how the ball would bounce off the rim given how it was shot. Then he'd have an advantage on securing the rebounds. He didn't have to do it. No one told him to. He was one of the best rebounders of all time. It takes what it takes.

Military example: General Patton defeated Rommel in Africa in tank warfare during World War II. One of Patton's keys to success during that campaign was that he read Rommel's German book on tank warfare. Patton was able to recognize Rommel's patterns and capitalize on them. Lives depended on Patton and Rommel, and Patton delivered because he had better knowledge. That only came from over-preparing.

Or consider a completely different pro example: There is a champion every year in the World Series of Poker. That sport is based solely on reading habits, body language, and a little luck. The same is true in other sports. Can you spot your opponent's body language and note when he's tired, when he's teetering and down? Can you see fear in them? You see a player's tendencies, then you know when to push and when not to. Take advantage and put him down.

Application: You play soccer. All right, can you kick equally well with your left and right side? No? Then you need to add that skill and elevate your game. Can you run and dribble with your head up to see the field? No? Fix it. Defend equally left and right? No? Fix it. Weak at "throw-ins"? Fix it. You're fast but not fast with the ball? Fix it. You turn the ball over? Fix it. Get pushed around because you're weak? Fix it. Ask your coach, what does an All-State or All-American or All-Pro player look like? Recognize and quantify the required skills and capabilities. Schedule the hours to home in on one until you have it. Then move onto the next one. Be Relentless.

Revisit the approach on Brainwashing. Recall what it is. I know you're on your phone. I know you're on it too much for you to be truly committed and Relentless to your targets and goals. All right, fine. Use it to your advantage. Line up podcasts, books on tape, or speeches that you can listen to. "Steal minutes" by listening to things in your car, while you're walking, working around your house and get better. If you play linebacker, then follow accounts on social media or YouTube videos about playing linebacker. You're on your phone anyway—use it to get better.

Remember, we improve what we measure. An easy example of a habit to implement is watching videos to improve yourself in your sport five times a week for at least twenty minutes (100 minutes total). Then schedule it. Then decide if you're a Pretender, College, Pro, or Statue kind of guy. Here is what that looks like: Pretender (<100 minutes), College (100 minutes), Pro (200 minutes), Statue (500+ minutes). Do this for two weeks and see where you're at. Decide if you need more, the same, or less. And then pick "more."

Here are some roadblocks: You don't know what you don't know. So ask! Who does know? Then whom do they listen to, read, watch videos on? Follow their habits. Tony Robbins says that "success leaves clues."

It's true. How about the most common roadblock: I don't have time. Honestly, from Jim Beebe's heart and mind: "You don't have time?!" For what you and I—we—are trying to do here, make the time, find the time, steal the time, whatever. Make it happen. And don't ever say that or think that again. You want to add something important to your life? Then you must remove something that is less important. Do it now. Why? You and I will be dead someday, and we only have one shot at what we want on Earth. So, we "got to go." *Now*!

CHAPTER 19

KNOWLEDGE - MENTORS

M entors. You must have them. At least one. "We grow taller by standing on the shoulders of giants." (No idea who said that, but it's true. Allegedly it was Bernard of Chartres.) What's that mean? It means that if you take a genius-level mathematician like Pythagoras or Euclid, I am way smarter than they were. And any high school kid that took calculus is way smarter too. Why? Pythagoras or Euclid never got to calculus. I did. So, I win. Isaac Newton discovered gravity, but I took three physics classes, so I beat him too. Not a big deal. There are tens of thousands beyond me. The phrase means that "giants" in any industry have all or most the knowledge in that industry during that time period. And others down the road study the giants and the greats and then get even smarter. The next generation evolved the information and gets even better at it. That's how it works. Think about it. The original automobiles had wood wheels. That was the best idea at the time. Yeah, well some cars today can go 200 mph. That's evolution.

Bill Belichick's father was the head football coach at the US Naval Academy. The Academy alone has several hundred books on football. Just football. In addition, Belichick was a huge Paul Brown fan who modernized and evolved the approach to coaching pro football well beyond his peers. Add in a lifetime of learning from the greats, plus all the books he read from other greats, plus his father and his contacts, and he's arguably the greatest football coach ever... for now. He took everyone else's knowledge and evolved it. Having a mentor, or two or more, simply increases the speed of your development. They learned years of lessons and now you can learn what they learned only faster. Mentors increase the speed at which you adapt and improve.

Actual Human Mentors

Working with and learning from people is optimal.

1. Talk face-to-face with people as much as possible. The mentor might have a simple idea or statement or habit to teach you. Let's say it's "Be Disciplined early every morning at 6:00 a.m. and set yourself up for success. Watch fifteen minutes of film to prepare your mind on your day's targets." The statement is helpful. It tells you when to start your day. It also tells you what to do each day. All good things. Then obvious questions arise: What is a good routine specifically? What if I have a 6:00 a.m. workout; does that mean I start at 5:00 a.m.? What changes when I travel for games, need more sleep, am on vacation, etc.? Now it's a conversation. Discuss the different ideas. It's two-sided too. On one side, you must stay Disciplined and do it daily. On the other side, there are always exceptions. Say Ball State just played in Toledo, Ohio on Tuesday night, and the team got on the bus to travel back to Muncie, Indiana and arrived back home to bed at 4:00 a.m.. It's not good for your morning routine to get up on two hours of sleep.

2. People form bonds with those they work with, identify with, and like. This happens a lot more with face-to-face encounters.

3. We are social creatures. Support is stronger together. Marriages don't work so well when spouses don't see each other for weeks or months at a time.

4. Want to know what your future looks like? Look at the five people you hang out with and work with the most.

Do-It-Yourself Mentors

1. Read. Period.
2. See Number 1 above. You can't be your best without getting smarter in your field. You also can't win without learning how to win at life. So, read. Read books, articles, etc. on how to get better mentally, nutritionally, in recovery—in short, the six Inch Blocks we outline here.
3. If you are looking for more specific help and training, contact us at Athlete Builder: www.athlete-builder.com or come to our gym to train and work with us in person: www.unbreakableathletic-sacademy.com.

On-Line Mentors

1. If you can't meet face-to-face, then meet online. Set up video chats and conferences. It's a small step below in-person meetings but still great. If not online, then have a phone conversation. Last resort is text and DMs. It's better than nothing. But so much is lost simply texting. You didn't come this far just to come this far. So, make your time count.
2. Not everyone worthwhile is nearby. My brother, Eric Beebe, is a very successful entrepreneur in Cleveland. We talk every Friday before lunch about how the week went. We hold each other accountable while we live in different states.
3. Some are masters of their craft and must be sought out. The only way to reach them is online. You get what you pay for too. So, find greatness and pay them for it. It's the same as paying Purdue University for a great engineering or business degree because Purdue is excellent. Find someone you need to learn the required skill from and hire them to mentor you.
4. Podcasts. There are excellent resources and discussions in podcasts. Revisit the Brainwashing section earlier in the book. You

love soccer? Listen to every podcast that has David Beckham or other soccer coaches on. Do this during your morning walk or while in the car. Maximize your time to get better.

5. Social media. The same authors, coaches, and podcasters have educational content on their social media pages. Absorb the free content and apply it. Move forward!

Systems of Mentors

For example, as my son Sam begins his senior year, he is considering playing soccer in college. I've always trained him for his Mindset and his strength and conditioning. Naturally, we discussed it. Then he talked with another D1 player I introduced him to at IUPUI, a local university. Then he talked with his current high school soccer coach. Finally, he talked with his former soccer coach as well. Sam has always been a joy to coach because he's so coachable and his effort is always through the roof. He took it upon himself to get as much information and data as possible to make his decision. He sought guidance from a number of great sources which helped a lot. As of this writing, he's looking at D3 and D2 schools if he wants to play. We will have to wait and see how his senior season unfolds and what he decides. But he has a plan and the help so he can make decisions and move forward.

1. It takes a village. What's the "one thing" I need to do to get better? I love Tim Grover's response: "There is never just one thing!" It's never as easy as one thing. Some things are more impactful than others, but it still takes dozens and hundreds of things to get better.

2. It takes multiple forms of mentorship to get better. The person who can teach you how to heal and recover isn't going to be the one to teach you how to train to become the strongest, fastest, most powerful athlete on the field. So, you need at least two.

3. You'll need all the forms listed above. You might need a book on recovery. You might listen to podcasts on mental toughness. You could meet with someone who is an expert at your sport and position. You might learn a ton on YouTube as well. It'll take many different forms.

4. Allies: It's easier and more effective to handle adversities together. We are talking about work here. Right? I'm asking you to think, decide, and act. So, find someone to act together with and you're more likely to stick to it.

5. Mindset: You need someone to help you advance and become mentally tougher. More resilient. Someone needs to push you to seek discomfort, to work. That's the only method for improving.

6. Knowledge: You need to become an expert in your craft. Who are potential mentors here? If you play linebacker, then start here: the starting linebacker, the starter who just graduated, your position coach, your defensive coordinator, All-State, All-Americans linebackers from your school, other high-level performers that you can reach out to. This last piece is a bit of a challenge. So, ask for help. Ask your position coach for a suggestion and an introduction.

7. Teammates. Who are the captains on your team? Work with them and see how they work and lead. Find someone in ROTC and meet with someone who's in a leadership role. Find out how they work with and lead others. You can't pick your family. And you can't pick your teammates. However, you will need to find a way to work with them so you can get where you want to go. It's better to find a way to work with them instead of against them.

8. Training. This is huge. Hopefully your S&C (strength and conditioning) coach is legit. Know this and tattoo it on your body and burn it into your brain. The best is near the top physically. That means close or near the top in strength, speed and power. Miss any of those components and you are not at the top and you are not at your own personal peak either. So, find someone to teach

you how to maximize those components. "Weak things break." – Louie Simmons. Be the strongest on the field and you have a legit shot.

1. I can get you strong, fast, and powerful. Period.

9. Nutrition. You must eat to perform. Someone needs to teach you. Two-thirds of any physical changes are a direct result of your Nutrition. You need a system. And your system will evolve as your season changes and as you age. There is no getting around it.

10. Recovery. You are putting yourself through hell to win. You must recover fast to do so. Again, you need to learn how. Find someone to teach you.

Process

Start with one. This book is a manual. Do *not* implement every strategy or tactic at once. It's overwhelming and not sustainable. Sustainability is far more important than being great just one time. It is so much more valuable to be very good consistently day in and day out, than it is to be great only occasionally.

Find one person to join your tribe and help you out. Connect with that person. Pick the primary area of focus. Most likely you will look for someone in your sport and work with that person. This is typically the primary target. However, it's not always the case. Look up Maurice Clarrett, the former one-hit-wonder running back for Ohio State. He was almost Heisman-worthy as a freshman and led his team to a national title. The NFL has a rule that athletes must be in college for three years prior to entering the draft. Well, Clarrett decided to challenge that rule. Long story short, he lost. He never played college football again, but he was still drafted after his three years were up. He went to the Denver Broncos and subsequently did not make the team. Fast forward a couple years, and he ended up in prison with an alcohol addiction.

Still, look him up. He completely turned his life around. He's a motivational speaker and travels the country helping kids out and getting them on the right path. He didn't need a football mentor. He needed a life skills mentor. That was his primary weakness. Now he's helping so many avoid the paths he chose. For yourself, find your biggest weakness, and find a mentor to help you through that challenge. Once you evolve and are working well with one mentor in your tribe, find another one for a different area. And repeat until you win everything.

Share your "Why." Be real. Be authentic. Be serious. Let your mentor know what you're after and why it's important. Why is it critical to you? Get deep into it. Then find more and more "Why's" that keep you on target in the same direction.

Work through your SWOT Analysis. Make your assessment of your SWOT Analysis and have your mentor do the same. Hopefully, he or she'll have meaningful insights as to other aspects you may not have realized. Remember the two main keys:

1. Your main strength is your competitive advantage. Constantly improve and elevate that area. It'll be the main way you beat others.
2. You must eliminate your main weaknesses at once. Be Relentless and crush it. This is the component that is holding you back the most.

Set Targets. Find the one habit that needs to occur that will further your competitive advantage. And find the one habit that must occur to fix your biggest weakness. Schedule it three to thirty times a week and execute. Write it down and track your results. Watch and see what happens. Example: a typical NFL receiver will catch two hundred balls from the jug machine daily. That is accomplished outside of practice. Their job is not to catch the easy balls coming their way. High school kids can do that. Their job is to catch every ball that comes their way, especially the bad ones. That's the extra margin that separates wins from losses, winners from losers, millions of dollars from being broke, Hall of Fame from not making the team.

Carrot and Stick. Reward and punishment. Accountability. Track your results daily. Get a notebook, a planner, or an app. Sure, there are the long-term rewards (having a long pro career) and punishments (getting cut from the team). Those are huge. However, it's the short-term consequences that lead to the long-term results. Collaborate with your mentor. Write down and share short-term rewards and punishments, and check in weekly on Fridays before noon. Example: Your optimal body fat to play at the pro level may be 9 percent. You're at 17 percent. Your three-month goal is to get to 14 percent. Your Nutrition targets and habits are set. Now you check in every thirty days to see if you're down 1 percent. You hit it? Great! Buy yourself new training swag. You miss it? Great! No swag. Do a walking lunge for one mile and adjust your habits and/or execution for the next month. You ever walk a lunge? I have. Normally DOMS (delayed onset muscle soreness) occurs a day or two later. I struggled to walk up the stairs from the soreness two hours later. You'll set a different, more realistic target next time. Or you'll execute like you should have in the first place and accomplish the goal.

Gratitude. No one must help anyone. No one. Others must choose to help or not. Think about it. I'm not helping you unless you buy the book. Otherwise, you probably don't know who I am. Your coaches are there to help. Your family could too. But to work with you one-on-one? That's time and effort. It's resources and money. And what goes around comes around. So be thankful and show them you're thankful. Help your mentor back. Reward and thank him. Be generous. He's changing your life! And when you can change someone else's, you'd better do it too. We're only on this planet once. Everything matters. Make your actions count. Be thankful and humble or you'll end up humbled.

The following people in these personal examples are all great people. They are not perfect. Don't expect that. It's unrealistic and a waste of time. But these people made an impact. They made me better.

Ed Bonchak: Unwavering ethics and Integrity. Always led me to be on a moral path. (I didn't always make the best choices, but I made a lot more because of Ed.) Ed went through a year of Catholic catechism so that when I needed a Catholic for my high school junior year Confirmation, he could do it. He's a police officer and a DARE officer for the Euclid Police Department.

Jay Hunt: Army Veteran. Head wrestling coach for John Hay High School in Cleveland. Taught me how to play racquetball which I ended up playing for Purdue University. On Saturdays for a summer, he and his wrestling team would take me on five-mile sandbag runs with "breaks" for hill sprints and calisthenics. When competing he taught me to add so much pain and pressure physically that my opponents would have to break before the match was over. Practice so hard the games would be easy. Jay passed in 2020, and I never talked with him after 1994. It's a regret.

Pete Dunbar: He started his own bank from scratch. Working for Pete in the banking world meant I had someone that knew every aspect of running a retail and commercial bank. That's unheard of. He is a true master of his craft. And every deal we put together for a client or prospect would save them money. Attention to detail and knowing every nuance was critical for our success. And it's fundamental to this day.

Eric Thomas, Tony Robbins, Jocko Willink. Podcasts, books, YouTube videos. You name it. Learn and apply. Learn and apply.

Instagram and social media: Eliminate crap. Follow sites that get you better. And move forward.

Atomic Habits, Legacy, The Way of the SEAL, Mastery, Awaken the Giant Within. Read everyone one of these books and more. But here's the thing. Read one at a time. Mark it up, highlight sections, take notes. Then it's time to move forward. Apply. Apply. Apply. Don't read a bunch of books and do nothing. What a huge mistake. Use your new knowledge to act.

Networking: Step 1, make people you meet better off. Hazel Walker with Business Network International taught me that lesson, and it's made all the difference. Introduce others to the people they are looking for. Make them smarter. Make them better. Then and only then should they start looking to do the same for you.

Toastmasters: If you want to speak, get around speakers. If you want to write, get around writers. Toastmasters help people speak better. Find a group that can help you with your craft. You make the all-star team? Great. Talk with those in your position and meet up to get better. Find the dawgs in your world and hang with them.

Eric Beebe: Survivor. Entrepreneur. Problem-solver. Sales guy. He can create something from nothing. He can lead from the front, middle, and back of the pack. He's a doer who finds the positive next step immediately. He's my youngest brother and my hero.

Jen Beebe: Wife, mother, powerlifter/strongwoman. She's great at systematically executing tasks. She gets hard tasks done daily because she's Relentless at doing the hard tasks first. She's also great at both Os in the OODA Loop military method (Observe and Orient). She takes in all the data and then decides. I go from "zero to sixty" quickly and sometimes act too hastily. I've had to learn those two great habits from Jen, but I still struggle to implement them as well as she does. Luckily, I have her on my side to help me.

CHAPTER 20

KNOWLEDGE - MINDSET

We already discussed Mindset previously. As a quick reminder, you don't know what you don't know. Fine. Now what? Your mentality is your Mindset. What path are you on? And why? Don't know? Go back and reread the Mindset section. It's okay. Happens all the time. Shoot, sometimes when I'm at Mass, I follow along with the reading that someone on the altar is reading aloud simultaneously. And sometimes my mind wanders (more than I'd like to admit). The reading ends and we move onto a song or a response, and I couldn't tell you at all what I just read. (Except of course the second reading was a letter from St. Paul. All the second readings are.) So, fine. I go back and reread it. Pay attention. And apply. Likewise, if you don't have the Knowledge to work on your Mindset, then go back and start that section over.

With each part of this book, the point is to do something. Move forward!

Your Mindset = movement = results = wins and losses (a.k.a. lessons).

Path 1: Mindset = fear and doubt = hesitation, resistance = lack of movement or weak movement = poor results = losses (lessons).

Path 2: Mindset = fear and doubt, but with resolve and Discipline despite that fear and doubt = steps forward = greater movement and increased confidence = better results = wins and still some losses (lessons).

Path 3: Mindset = resolve and Discipline, but with Relentless tenacity = giant leaps forward and dragging Teammates with you = enormous movement and increased confidence = best results = greater wins and still some losses (lessons).

Keep evolving your path. Confidence only comes from reps. You must learn how to change, improve, and evolve your Mindset. There is no need to rehash the steps in this section. The prior chapters on Mindset have covered it. The point here is that, again, you'll need increased Knowledge in the six Blocks. Just when you think you have all the answers, you'll realize that you have more questions than answers. If you want to achieve new heights, ask bigger and harder questions. The answers to those questions will help formulate a road map of what your next steps should be. Then you must decide "the ONE thing" (Keller) that will advance you the furthest and then "prioritize and execute" (Willink). Just Do It (Nike).

CHAPTER 21

KNOWLEDGE - TEAMMATES

This information you're reading is just in a book. What you learn in school is great too, but again it's merely in a classroom setting. ("Don't let your schoolwork get in the way of your education." – Mark Twain.) Similarly, what your coaches teach you in film study and on the practice field are just that: practice. Greatness comes from learning all and learning more, and most of all how you apply it.

Military example: OODA Loop

- Observe: Collect as much data as possible using all your senses.
- Orient: Analyze the data and map out everything as best you can.
- Decide: You must pick your best course of action. This is not the perfect course of action, but the best. Even if your probability for success is 51 percent for and 49 percent against, pick the 51 percent.
- Act: Yes, again your brain must make you act. Move Forward. And start the process over. Mike Tyson always says, "Everyone has a plan until they get hit in the face." Keep the Loop going and evolve more quickly than everyone else.

We will discuss the Knowledge component in detail in its own section. The point here is that you must take time and measures to learn more about how to work with others. Here are some of the basics of what you must learn with Teammates:

Coaches

You have no shot if you cannot learn to work with your coaches. Yes, you must learn their game plans and schemes. That's obvious. But you also must learn how they want them implemented. The "what" and the "how" go together. You must learn them both. You must also learn the subtleties and tactics of communicating with your coach. Learn to be aware of his moods and tendencies. Timing will be everything.

Here's a high-level approach: Learn the playbook and commit it to memory. (Obvious.) Learn the changes to this week's game plan. (Also obvious). Then learn what the coach would want with contingencies. What four to six main contingencies would he want you to know if certain scenarios unfolded on the field? Learn that too! (Not obvious) Then you can elevate yourself to a quasi-coach on the field. This will naturally elevate your performance and the team's. How do you get there? Ask. (Obvious.) "Hey Coach, what are two or three things that worry you that the other team might do to counter our approach? What should I look for? Then what should I do when I see that?" Then do that.

Players/Teammates

You ever watch the football movie, *Any Given Sunday*? "Steamin'" Willie Beamon told ESPN and the press that the team's success was solely attributable to his own play. No one else helped or was responsible. Beamon was the QB for Miami's football team, the Sharks. Beamon said the defense wasn't up to his standards of play. The offensive line wasn't good enough either. Well, the next game, the weather was an enormous factor because of the wind and rain. Beamon's offensive line decided not to block very well that game, and Beamon was left hurting from head to toe and with a loss for the game. Can you get along with your teammates? You must learn how others interact with you and the team as well. You must also learn how you must interact with them. What is your process for interacting when you're not playing well or feeling down? What do you do when your Teammate feels the same way? How do you adjust? Keep notes in your notebook or journal.

Here is an example at Unbreakable Athletics. I was coaching two different females in a CrossFit session. They were similar in age and both technically proficient, but totally different in personality and competitiveness. Arien was working on her snatch (an Olympic lift) and adding weight up to a one rep max. I had her add only the smallest of increments (5 lb. each lift) as she advanced. I'd say, "I'm not sure yet about hitting your PR (personal record) number yet today. But I'm totally sure that if we only add 5 lb. more to the next set that it's a lock. It's guaranteed." Then she'd hit that set and do it well. The next set, she added five more pounds and continued in that fashion. After so many sets, it was hard to keep track of the total. She continued up the ladder and eventually PR'd that day. Great! I kept her focused on the fact we only added five pounds and not the total. ("Where focus goes, energy flows." – Tony Robbins.) It kept her calm and confident, and she performed better because of it.

Later that day, Sarah came in to snatch for her training session. At the time, her PR was very similar to Arien's. All I had to do was say what Arien snatched that day, and Sarah would respond, "Oh, I'm going to hit that number and pass her, then." I merely had to give her a target and told her what her competitor did, and she was off and running. For Arien, I had to bring her along more slowly and systematically. Both achieved the same result, a PR. Both had two different routes to it, though.

You must do the same thing. Try to get as much out of your Teammates as possible. Each is different. And the team's roster changes a lot every year. The good thing is that you're not the head coach yet. Don't try to be. That's not your job. Start small with your main circle of friends on the team. Push each other to excel. Push hard. Get your "tribe" working, training, and fighting for the same thing. Then see if you can expand to your position group. If you can improve your knowledge of how to affect those two groups, you'll be ahead of the next guy.

Here is a quick three-step process for doing so:

1. Be authentic and real. Simply say what you want. ("I want to win. I want to win a conference title. I want to dominate and be named all-conference." Just be real.)
2. Over-communicate with your Teammates involved. Let them know and ask for help.
3. Focus on working together. Ask a Teammate to do extra work with you.

Leading

Always start leading by example. Be firm but humble. Do more than everyone else to build credibility. Own all shortcomings and mistakes. Keep at it with your best effort. It's like parenting. If you "give a shit," then you'll be okay. Why? Because you care enough to do your best and care for the group before you care for yourself.

Talk with the coaches and the captain (if you aren't one yet) and ask what they need from you. Take their direction to heart and over-execute your assigned tasks. Keep taking notes and learning.

A sound process is this:

• Learn to lead by example first: Be the first one to meetings and the facility to train. Last one to leave, too. "Champions do more" work. So do it.

- Learn how to lead your roommates or people at your same position. If you're not the best or smartest in your immediate group, then you must learn to lead with attitude and effort.
- Once you're an "expert" at your position, then it's game on. Get everyone around you better. You must continue with your earlier steps in the process: attitude, effort, example, but then add in your Knowledge and what the coaches and captains want.
- If you don't know how or what to do? Ask! Read! Learn! A million people have done it before you came along. Find someone and get their Knowledge so you can evolve faster.
- Consistency matters. Always and forever. Consistency builds credibility. You must do this daily.

Support Group

This is a lifelong endeavor to learn. You must learn how to work within your family and friends. And that group changes. In high school, your family leaders are most likely your parents. In college, they are not nearly as much. After college, it could be a significant other/spouse and then potentially kids. That's just your life on your family's side. Luckily, the main consistency in families is how universally dysfunctional we all are. That's a "fun" wrinkle in the mix.

Be very careful in your close circle of friends. The true ones. . . man, they are rare. Learn to give first before asking. Learn to set clear boundaries. Then learn to enforce them. If you can learn to be at peace when you're alone, then you won't have the fears of walking away from toxic or debilitating relationships. You'll need to learn this is necessary for you to advance as far as you can go.

Allies

This is huge. And it's typically not family members and friends. But it could be. Your ally is one person or a group of Teammates, on or off the field. This is the group with the same singular focus and resolve to advance. It's win at all costs with you and this group. Learn you need three or four in this group to crush the competition. Choose wisely and take your time when selecting allies. In business, the mantra is "Hire slowly and fire quickly." It's true. And it works.

Resources

Learn what your trainers must know to help you. What must you learn to do on your own from them and apply yourself? Example: Sarah with Myo-Fit in Indianapolis is hands down excellent. Myo-Fit is her company. She's also the head athletic trainer with a master's degree. I've known her for more than ten years. She's an expert and provides expert service. I had to learn the basics from her on how my body worked relative to what I was doing to train. I have poor internal hip rotation. (Everything impacts everything.) My hips impacted my walking gait. My gait impacted my lower back. Normally, who cares? Walking is walking, and it's hard to get hurt simply from that. But in a strongman competition when I'm asked to carry a 700+ lb. yoke, a 300+ lb. Husafell stone, and 300 lb./hand farmers carry, then my low back, gait, hips (everything!) must be moving correctly, or I won't just lose. I'll get extremely hurt. Sarah had to teach me about that. Then she would work on me. And finally, she would have to teach me my "homework" so I could continue to move better when she was done. Of course, doing the homework is not a Knowledge thing; it's a Discipline thing. But Knowledge was huge for me to survive in that sport.

CHAPTER 22

KNOWLEDGE - THREE MUST KNOW BASICS

Some make a career in a small component that deals with the human body. You'll need to get the basics in a multitude of areas to optimize your performance as an athlete. It must be learned. Your Knowledge in the different areas must increase if you have any hopes of winning. (Recall the "no chance" percentage. You must make it to the top.) Knowledge is most certainly power.

Also keep in mind that I am giving you some of the basics that will absolutely help you. However, it is as important that you learn what you need and how your body responds to actions.

Some of you might be able to go out drinking during the week of a game and still perform well. Well, your ability to do so is dramatically different when you're twenty-one versus thirty years old. You'll need to learn how your body processes things. And in all reality, if you're going out drinking the week of a big game, you don't have "it." You don't have what it takes to be the best version of you. But the point here is that you will need to learn to adjust your approach to things. And every few years, you'll have to relearn it because your body will age and change. Again, your circumstances also will change (e.g., going from only playing some on JV to playing a lot on varsity to playing a lot in the pros).

Another example: Your body recovers quickly from football practice in high school. You'll quickly learn that adding ice baths after football practice in college isn't only a suggestion but a requirement for your body to heal up from the increased workload. You'll need more in the pros too, obviously. But what if you're "the man": Michael Jordan, Kobe Bryant, Ray Lewis, Tom Brady, Aaron Judge, etc.? Then the load is even greater because you carry most of the stress and most of the work. Again, Knowledge is power.

The Body

Don't forget, we are discussing the following three topics (Training, Nutrition, and Recovery) fully in their own sections. Just realize and recognize that you must increase your Knowledge in each area.

Success leaves clues. Heck, success leaves a roadmap (this book, other books, other athletes, coaches, etc.) and habits that scream at you. Just find the answers. Who plays your position well at a prominent level in your area? What's that mean? For example, you play center back in soccer in high school. Who else plays center back in high school soccer and is all-state or the best in the state? Who played the same position and went on to play D1 soccer from the prior two to three years? All right, now let's figure it out.

- What was their size and shape typically? Body fat percentage?
- How was their speed, strength, and stamina in a game and over a season?
- What made them physically superior? That's the real question.

Now get to those measurables and a little bit beyond.

Training

- Learn what physical tools you'll need. Leg strength. Core strength. Strong quads to kick the ball far and hard and sprint fast. Strong hamstrings to balance out your quads and help against ACL tears.
- Strong torso to help protect you against collisions and set your body up for maximal output.
- Elite-level speed to separate yourself from the competition.
- Strong neck to help protect you against concussions and falls.
- Elite-level reflexes with eye-foot coordination.
- Follow this progression. It's a law. Follow laws and win. (I wish I made the laws, but alas, I do not. But I do work the laws to death. Like $F = M \times A$. Force = Mass × Acceleration.)
  - Nutrition → Move correctly and consistently → GPP (General Physical Preparedness) → Strength → Power and speed → Sport-specific skills. Let's clarify. To be healthy, the most important base starts with Nutrition. Then you must learn to move correctly and consistently. After that, it's more important to be "in shape," which comes from GPP. From there you want to add strength to your body. Once you're strong, it's very easy to get faster and more powerful. The last step is to improve at your sport. This is the order of priorities to become healthy. You are simply taking it to the next level to become the best athlete you possibly can.
  - Example of a world of negligent coaches who get it horribly wrong: coaches on fourteen-year-old softball/baseball teams working kids for ten to eleven months a year on baseball-specific skills. Meanwhile, the kids are out of shape. The kids can't hit the ball out of the infield because they are criminally weak. And they aren't powerful or fast. Result: weak kids with shoulder injuries and burnout who overall

are not athletic. Answer: Take a few days less to practice and add strength and conditioning to make resilient athletes.

- Set up your training to make this happen. Your school strength and conditioning coach can get you part of the way there. It's fifty-fifty they are good at what they do, have the capacity because of coaching, time, and equipment constraints. Answer: champions do more. Find another coach or mentor and ask what it takes to win physically and move forward. Follow the progression listed above. Get in shape. Move your body weight perfectly. Get strong as needed to be elite in your sport (Meaning if you are a 2–2.5× bodyweight squatter, then you have enough leg strength to be legit in soccer. No need to add more strength.) Next, get as fast and as powerful as humanly possible in your sport. Huge separator here! Last, use your superior physical capabilities to perfect your craft in your individual skills.

Nutrition

I'll give you the basics here. But what you really need to learn is how you and your body react to the basics. Then you'll also need to reevaluate how you and your body react to the basics at different periods in your life. Obvious example: Your metabolism will change as you age, as you are typically less active, as you have less muscle, and how well you recover or don't recover changes.

How? Take notes and keep them. Write your own playbook. Then adjust. Adapt.

Here are the priorities. Don't move onto a step until the prior one is a legit habit.

1. Stop eating like a true idiot. You know what I mean. You know who you are and what you do. Stop it.
2. Track what you eat. We improve what we measure. We can't change or improve a habit until we have it. So, we need to know what you're eating. Notebook, journal, phone/table notes, etc. I like the app My Fitness Pal.
3. Learn the basics of nutrition: calories, carbohydrates, fats, proteins, water. (This will occur in the Nutrition section of this book.)
4. Consume between 0.75–1.25 times your bodyweight in grams of protein depending on needs and desires. So, if you weigh 160 lb., then consume 120–200 g of protein/day.
5. Set your calories to keep you at a body fat percentage that is optimal for your sport's performance.
6. Start with 5–6 g of creatine daily. After three to four months, move to 10 g and stay there.
7. Take in a good probiotic and fish oil.
8. Consume as much fruit and vegetables as you can.

Recovery

Just like Nutrition, I'll give you the basics. Here is the main thing: It's not how hard or intense you can work, train, compete, etc. It's not. It's how hard or intense can you train *and* recover *and* train again. I can bring in an athlete and smash them on Monday. Then they can't get "smashed" again until probably Thursday. At a minimum, the athlete cannot be that intense on Tuesday or Wednesday (maybe 60–70 percent of potential). But either way, they won't be able to be intense again until later in the week. And the law: Intensity = Results. So now what? Answer: Be as intense in your training as your recovery allows you to be.

Here is another thing to look at with intensity/recovery. Sometimes you are shot. Your CNS (central nervous system) is wrecked. You don't feel like doing much of anything. And you want to take a zero in your training. You want to quit that day. (Don't do it. Sisu is a Core Value!) Well, you can't be intense. You can't really be moderately intense. But you can come in and move. Work on some mobility. Get blood flowing with some basic conditioning and lifting and, metaphorically, score a 50 percent. Well, 50 percent is a failing grade for sure. But what does a 0 percent look like? So, if there are three days a month when you are supposed to train but feel wrecked, just get a 50 percent score. If I do that and get 150 percent (3 × 50 percent) for those three days and you get 3 × 0. I win.

Just like Nutrition, you'll need to learn what you need to do to recover. This process will evolve too (e.g., as you add more work, experience stressors in your life, and age). Yes, you guessed it. Take notes. Be Relentless!

Priorities. Do These In Order.

1. Sleep is the number one steroid. Hands down. Learn how to maximize this.
2. Water is a must. Muscles need it. Creatine holds it in the muscles. Drink your water. How much? Enough so that your urine throughout the day is like light lemonade in color.
3. Do your own body treatments: rolling, ice baths, mobility/stability work.
4. Meditate. Learn how to calm your mind.
5. Get treatments from your trainers, chiropractors, massage therapists, etc.
6. Take your supplements (kind of a Nutrition thing here, but it aids recovery too).
7. When in doubt, repeat Step 1.

CHAPTER 23

KNOWLEDGE - WAY OF INCHES

Time to move forward. Time to act. To be clear, think about your Knowledge in terms of being the athlete that you are. Don't think about your Mindset, your Training, or any of the other six Blocks in this section. Focus solely on your Knowledge needed to play your sport during an actual game, at an elite level. That's it. Yes, all other Blocks affect your performance. For this part of your performance, focus solely on your skills and Knowledge in your sport. The following is the Inches Way: Knowledge section of the Assessment Test:

KNOWLEDGE

Playbook (Points are doubled here because of their significance.)

- 10 Points: You know your critical skills, your position's duties, your unit's duties, your offense's or defense's duties, and your opponents' duties perfectly.
- 8 Points: You know all skills and duties for your position, unit, and your offense or defense.
- 7 Points: You know all skills and duties for your position and unit.
- 6 Points: You know all skills and duties for your position.

- 0 Points: You do not know your position skills and duties perfectly.

POINTS: _____

This is the same score as the last question above. That's how valuable it is

Life

- 10 Points: You have a plan and process to manage your critical life skills now and for the future for you to perform at your best in your sport.
- 7 Points: You are getting by day-to-day, and it affects your play.
- 2 Points: Your environment (clutter, cleanliness, paying bills, etc.) at home is in disarray.

POINTS: _____

Kaizen

- 10 Points: You have a process for improving and adhere to it without fail.
- 8 Points: You mostly have a process and adhere to it.
- 5 Points: You occasionally have a process and adhere to it.
- 0 Points: All else.

POINTS: _____

Knowledge Mentor

- 10 Points: You have one and connect weekly.
- 8 Points: You have one and connect monthly.
- 5 Points: You have one and connect quarterly.
- 0 Points: All else.

POINTS: _____

How effectively are you working with a Knowledge accountability ally (or allies)?

- 10 Points: You and your ally review your results weekly, enforce a "carrot/stick," and adjust.
- 7 Points: You and your ally review your results monthly and sometimes enforce "carrot/stick."
- 4 Points: You and your ally review your results quarterly.
- 0 Points: All else.

POINTS: _____

You know your number one Knowledge Strength (Competitive Advantage):

- 10 points. Otherwise: 0 points.

POINTS: _____

You know your number one Knowledge Weakness (Weak Link):

• 10 points. Otherwise: 0 points.

POINTS: _____

You know your number one Knowledge Opportunity (Target):

• 10 points. Otherwise: 0 points.

POINTS: _____

You know your number one Knowledge Threat (Enemy):

• 10 points. Otherwise: 0 points.

POINTS: _____

TOTAL POINTS: _____

OVERALL AVERAGE (TOTAL POINTS / 10) _____

You see your score. Retest yourself at the end of every quarter of the year (March 31, June 30, September 30, December 31).

Here we go again. Ask yourself a series of reflective questions and gauge your progress over the last quarter.

• What's your level of Knowledge of the playbook? More importantly what is your level of Knowledge for playing your position at the highest level? How did you progress/regress over that last ninety days? We care more about the direction than we do about where you are at currently. Meaning, it's more important that you're working to improve consistently than it is where you are right now.

- What's your level of Knowledge of the other positions on your team so you can lead them the field? What is your level of Knowledge of the players and how they perform so you can motivate and get the most out of them as well?
- What's your level of Knowledge of the teams on your schedule? Personnel, strengths, weaknesses, and tendencies?
- What's your level of life skill Knowledge?

SWOT analysis. This time apply your SWOT analysis to the Knowledge Block not Mindset. Be sure to prioritize and identify your Competitive Advantage and your Weak Link. You must advance in these areas to perfect your performance. Write out your process goals and habits for the next quarter. What is your number one Target for this quarter? Share with your Knowledge accountability ally. Devise your carrot and stick for your check-ins. Bring on a mentor as well. I can't imagine a scenario where you work this diligently and don't advance. It's impossible. You'll continue to crush it.

- Strength:
    ◦ List them all.
    ◦ What are your top three?
    ◦ What is your number one Strength (Competitive Advantage)?
- Weaknesses:
    ◦ List them all.
    ◦ What are your top three?
    ◦ What is your number one Weakness (Weak Link)?
- Opportunities:
    ◦ List them all.
    ◦ What are your top three?

- What is your number one Opportunity (Target)?
- Threats:
  - List them all.
  - What are your top three?
  - What is your number one Threat (Enemy)?

Knowledge Way of Inches

Where do you want to be at the end of "this section" of your career in terms of Knowledge? Note: If you're in high school, then "this section" of your career is at the end of your senior season. In college, it's the end of your college senior season. As a pro, it's your retirement day. Back that up. Where do you want to be at the end of the next season? Back it up again. Where do you want to be in a month? In a week? Tomorrow?

Based on your answers above and your SWOT analysis, what is today's Inch Challenge?

What days and times this week will you work on your Knowledge Inch Challenge? Each hour worked on it gains you a Knowledge Inch. Win a Knowledge Inch and win the day. Two Knowledge Inches are better than one Knowledge Inch. Keep building. Keep winning.

What are the obstacles that get in the way? List them. These are the threats, your opponent, your enemy. Remember, you still need an Inch, so you need a solution to your obstacle. One day, you get thirty minutes of work done on your Knowledge Inch because it's Christmas, and you're with your family. Great! Half of an Inch is better than no Inch. Win!

At the end of your week, tally up your score. See how you did versus your plan. Give yourself the carrot or stick. And then revise your plan for next week. Wash, rinse, repeat. Attack, attack, attack. Win, win, win! Sustainability is the goal. It is not one momentous day each month. Get a little bit better daily and build your Blocks. See how much larger you can build yourself, and your Inch building blocks will show it.

10 Knowledge Habits

Not sure exactly what to do? Need ideas? Do these. Remember, pick one at a time and execute. No, over-execute. Don't do it until you get it right. Do it until you can't get it wrong. Remember the push-ups and Statue > Pro Athlete > College Athlete > Pretender.

1. Be the supreme leader in the playbook for the team. Critical. Take the amount of time you spend studying the playbook each day and triple it.
2. Continue step one until you know your "side of the ball" (offense or defense) and become the supreme leader in the playbook for the team.
3. Practice for forty-five minutes every day after the standard team practice to learn more skills. My son Sam always had a ball with him and would work on his soccer moves daily and then drop them in practices and games.
4. Arrive twenty minutes prior to team and position meetings armed with two questions on what to learn next or to get better.
5. Read ten pages or for thirty minutes daily to learn more on your craft or sport. You must be a student of your sport to understand all of its intricacies and master it.
6. Ask your mentor what to learn and read next. Schedule two hours a week to work on it.
7. Keep a training and game log. Learn what you need to do to prepare for each. Learn what you need to do when practicing and playing in different weather, when behind on sleep, etc. Write down your notes so you know how to perform better next time.
8. Master one "move" you can do at any time in your life on the field or court. This "move" is one you can execute perfectly, even with a 103-degree fever while vomiting from the flu. Once you

have your "move," then develop a second one. And repeat. Relentlessly.

9. Talk with other "greats" in your sport past and present. Don't know any? Ask your coach for a referral or suggestion. Regularly discuss different ideas and nuances. Take notes. Try out new things and experiment. Continue to evolve.

10. Teach what you learn to your teammates. If you can teach a concept, then you must truly know it.

Scan the following QR code or visit: https://athlete-builder.com to access and download the assessment in this chapter and other resources (free nutrition resources and free workout programs).

CHAPTER 24

TEAMMATES

L et's be crystal clear. In this instance, in this book, Teammates are simply anyone and everyone you work with to achieve something, anything. This topic of discussion also falls under the "Head" Block because you interact with people verbally. It's not really a physical skill.

Now, know this: No one gets anywhere alone. No one. Ever. Do you do most of your work alone? Yes, absolutely. When you compete, a lot of the outcome is "on you." You must own everything. Did you do everything? Nope. Can you? No chance. This means the art and science of working with others becomes necessary.

What about. . . ?

- "I live alone. No one helps me." You have a coach and teammates on the court or field.
- "I play golf. I'm alone." You have a caddy and a coach.
- "I'm a bowler." Someone taught you how to bowl.
- "I don't like people." Quit now. You won't get far by yourself.
- "I'm all alone." There are no atheists in foxholes. God is with you. (What's a foxhole? It's a self-dug hole for you to hide in while the enemy army is launching bombs at you.)

No one does it alone.

Many, many books are written about getting along with and working with others. We need to work out a process for you to become the best athlete you can be. Let's discuss you, yourself, first.

Banker Face

I've worked in banking, finance, investments, and white-collar crime for fifteen years prior to changing to strength and conditioning with my gym. It was my "first life" out of college and getting my master's degree from Purdue University. When I was dealing with the public, customers, or even coworkers, sometimes I needed my "banker face" on. Banker face means I don't always say what I think and feel. Could you imagine walking around speaking every thought you had? Sometimes you need to keep thoughts to yourself. Sometimes you don't.

First, in any instance or relationship, you must make your own assessments and evaluations. You'll need to do this with people as well as circumstances. Next, you must decide how you want to interact and communicate during those times. Take a moment and be careful here. Your next steps will determine your future. You're working with people for you to play sports at a high level.

Example: You play football, and you want more playing time as you're working your way up the depth chart. "Hey dumbass, why aren't you playing me?!" Or "Coach, can I get ten minutes with you? I'm trying to improve so I can play and help us win. I have two questions." The difference is obvious. Discipline is how you handle that situation. Discipline also determines your fate in this instance.

Keep your thoughts to yourself until the time when opening your mouth furthers your cause and the cause of your team. There is no need to push a situation with anyone until it's necessary. All the while, you must be aware of how you're interacting with your team. You must recognize how the coaches work with you. The same is true with the support staff. Your support staff includes those associated with your team and your personal relationship as well.

Temet nosce. Know thyself. You must be true to yourself. Honest and authentic. Be real and objective with your thoughts. Once you have something to contribute to your team, then speak up, speak loudly, speak often. Get in the discussions and make an impact with others around.

Sponge

Soak up everything. Elite-level coaches in the NFL are fired annually. Each has ten thousand hours and more required to be true masters of their craft. By age thirty-five, most have already been in the game for three decades. What's this mean to you? Your road to expert-level Knowledge is long ahead of you. Show up early for every meeting and ask questions? Talk to everyone. Learn every minute detail and nuance to your sport and craft. It'll take your entire career to become an expert. Start now.

"Success leaves clues." – Tony Robbins. Thousands of people have come before you in your sport. You'll need to work with everyone to soak up their knowledge and get up to speed with the rest of the world.

How do you do this? Ask. Be authentic. And then ask again. Apply what you learned. And then update that person with your progress. In each instance, be humble and thankful.

Personal example: It was January of 2009. The US was in another financial crisis, this time the housing bubble. I had one semester left at Purdue finishing up my master's in finance. Think about that: master's in finance during a financial crisis. It was a terrible time to look for a job. Normally the job-placement rate upon graduation was well above 90 percent. My class "enjoyed" a rate of around 24 percent. With a mountain of student loans and three kids (huge "sticks"), I had to have a job upon graduation. I got one at the largest bank in the country, JP Morgan Chase. How?

I was studying around midnight in Rawls Hall, the MBA building. Kevin, an undergraduate, was studying at the table next to me. I'd never met him before. At one point, I took a break and turned to him. "What are you working on?"

Kevin responded, "Statistics."

"Me too." It was just that I was doing graduate-level work while he was doing undergraduate-level work. He was struggling with his work, and I checked it out. It was a type of combination problem. I looked at his work and noticed he wasn't using a formula that would have made all his work much easier.

So, I pointed that out. "Why don't you use this formula?"

Kevin said, "We haven't learned that yet."

"Oh. Whoops. Well, looks like you will next week. If you use the formula now, your work will be much easier."

"Thanks! I'll give it a shot. Appreciate it. I'm Kevin."

From there, I introduced myself and we got to talking. We let each other know what we were looking to do after graduation. He asked, "Well, if you want to work in finance in Indianapolis, then would you like to meet someone who works in private equity?"

"Hell yeah!" Private equity work is the holy grail in the finance world. Kevin emailed his cousin David to introduce me. Next, I forwarded him my résumé and asked for fifteen minutes to learn more about him, his company, and the industry. After meeting with him, he sent me to another private equity guy, Faraz. I did the same thing here: emailed Faraz the résumé and asked for fifteen minutes to learn more about him, his company, and the industry. Then I let David know how the meeting went with Faraz and thank David again. My next meeting with Faraz went well again. During that meeting, Faraz suggested I attend the Venture Club of Indianapolis. This club brings together entrepreneurs, investors, lawyers, bankers, accountants, students, and more. Perfect. It would be an entire room of people available for more fifteen-minute appointment sessions with me.

Next thing I knew, I was at the Venture Club. Faraz introduced me to someone there, who introduced me to someone else. Then I was introduced to Lynette. She worked in the high-level private bank within

JP Morgan Chase. BAM! Lynette and I got to talking. JP was already hiring during the financial crisis and was looking for someone with experience. Long story longer, I got the job when I graduated in May.

Lessons: Always conduct yourself well. Make solid relationships. Be real and authentic. Help others first. And what goes around will come around.

Painful lesson: I was the head of financial investigations at the Indiana Gaming Commission. This spanned a little over three years right before I returned to Purdue for my master's. My prior places of employment were in financial institutions. I was a broker and a lender. My groups mostly were all-male and had a "locker room" culture where we were hunting for sales. Let's just say that working for the Gaming Commission and the State of Indiana was. . . different. As it should be

The CFO had made a small error and it was costing me time and efforts within my division. Great solution: Set up twenty minutes to discuss the matter and resolve the issue and the slow process. My moronic solution: Send an email pointing out the CFO's failures and missteps and that I had to problem-solve for the CFO. Result: My boss needed a meeting with me to get me straightened out and acting like a grown-up and a professional. Then I needed to apologize sincerely and eat it. Honestly, I truly deserved it. Lesson: Don't be an idiot like I was.

On your team, Tim Grover says it's better to be feared than liked. It's true. Respect is valued over common friendships when it comes to performing well and winning. Move silently along until it's time to speak up. Actions always speak loudest. Your ability to execute is what inspires others. It's what the coaches notice. It's the only way to advance. Look around; watch and see. The loudest people are loud because they are compensating. Be so great so you can't be ignored. I told my sons, Jack and Sam, their job was to earn Coach of the Year awards for their head coach based on their play. Otherwise, get the coach fired for being so stupid for not playing them. Both instances could only occur if his play was the best in the state. When you can execute at the highest level, respect is a given. Your words will carry the most weight then. Does that mean never to speak up until then? Of course not. But make sure when you open your mouth, it's improving the situation and the team. Have the conversations come from a good place.

Use the eye test. You communicate with your Teammates and coaches through everything you do. Actions > Words. Words are not silent. How you dress matters. Punctuality matters. Where you sit in team meetings matters. Effort screams! Professionalism screams! Your persona and how you carry yourself make an impact. You should know this by now. Take yourself out of sports for a second. You're at a team party at someone's house. You're talking to someone of the opposite sex. Can you tell if he or she is interested in you? Yup, sure can. Can you tell if he or she is *not* interested in you? Yup, sure can. Body language screams!

Say you're new to the team in college. You're not getting many reps at all because you're a walk-on. Where can you win? Where can you set yourself apart? Where can you make an impact? Everywhere!

You can. . .

- Be the hardest worker in the weight room. Lead by example. You'll create the culture necessary for your team to win.
- Be the most supportive athlete in the weight room.
- Be the first one to team meetings by thirty minutes. And you have a specific question you need answered so you can improve, each day.
- Be the last one to leave the meetings. Of course, you sit in the front row, too.
- Meet with the trainers to learn the little things you can do to heal faster once you're banged up. Learn to work with your support staff.
- Ask the coach for two skills you must perfect to advance. Hammer those immediately to perfection. It's not that you got it right.

It's that you can't get it wrong. Then it's back to the coach to let him know and get the next level of work.

- Ask a team captain how you can help.
- Have the highest GPA. Show that achieving high standards in the classroom and in your sport are doable.
- Watch an extra ninety minutes of film each day. Pass your new knowledge on to your Teammates.
- Keep your room, your locker, your car in order. Are you a Pretender that couldn't get to the minimum twenty-five push-ups? Or are you the guy that does fifty without blinking? Being Disciplined also helps impact your team culture.
- Find a mentor! Squeeze every ounce of information from him to improve. Thank him profusely. And get another one.

If you're a walk-on, then prep, work, and carry yourself like a starter. If you're a starter, conduct your business like you're a captain. Captain? Great—lead that team to a championship and run your life like you're All-State or All-American. Keep pushing. Get to that Statue level where people notice. Everyone is trying to emulate and catch up to your level and work ethic. Become unbreakable.

CHAPTER 25

TEAMMATES - YOUR SQUAD

"You want to see a glimpse of your future? Show me the five people you hang out with most." – Jim Rohn

"If you walk with the lame, you'll develop a limp." – Louie Simmons

"The strength of the pack is the wolf. And the strength of the wolf is the pack." – Rudyard Kipling

That's the deal. If you can apply those rules well, you've got it. If not, then you have work to do. Your goal: Get your team better. Get them a lot better. If you do that, then what happens? Competition improves. It gets harder. Then if you want to play and be able to hang with your team, then you must also improve. Otherwise, you'll get left behind.

Here is where Integrity arrives. Human behavior says, don't get your team better. If you're a point guard on your team, don't get your backup better. Don't get the other point guard better. Why? Because you could lose your job. Why else? Because you'll have to work more, evolve more, learn more to keep your job. It will take more effort. Not pushing others because you will have to push as well is a weak mindset. Rise above that lower level.

We are grooming winners. Strong-minded warriors who seek discomfort to push forward. If you're on a team, then the goal is to win. Win often. And win the big games. So, get your teammates better. Now.

Training example: At my strongest, I deadlifted 600+ lb. three times in my life. It took me eight years to get there from age thirty-seven to forty-five. Each of those lifts were witnessed by Training partners who were seasoned and experienced. They knew me and how I trained and lifted. They were strong, too, and pushed me while I pushed them. When you're "laddering up" in a lift, you add weight each set until you're at the desired weight for the day. As it gets heavier and harder, it gets slower and more painful. You can't see your own lift or the speed and form. But your partners can. They can look for mistakes and breakdowns. They can cue you to move more efficiently. They can witness the speed as well. All those points help assess and evaluate the day's training.

It also helps to have others "call" your next weight as you ladder up. An objective Teammate is critical to have when training to your max potential. My first time pulling over six hundred pounds was at the Rathskeller during German Fest. We were doing a Bavarian deadlift during the festival. My wife is an excellent, objective coach for me. I had just pulled 508 and she called 558 next for me. Those 558 lb. went up decently, but it was not blazing fast. In my mind it "felt" slow, but how would I know? I'm biased and couldn't see the lift. So I asked her what the call was. She said, "Call for 608. It'll be a slow grind, but pull for a minimum of four to six seconds. And ask that big dude behind you to spot you." (The "big dude" was Robert Knutsson @bigsweed87 on Instagram. He's a great athlete and powerlifter. He's a tank!) It was my turn to lift. I dialed in, set my back and lats. I used an over/under grip and hook grip as well. I started pulling, and it was very slow going. It was taking forever, and my vision was starting to go dark. It seemed like I was looking through a tube and the tube was shrinking. I was starting to black out from holding my air and pressure. The judge had his arm up for my down command. At the halfway point, I knew to squeeze my butt with everything I had. I locked out the lift and received my down command. I put the weight down and started to buckle. Robert had his hand in the back of my belt so I wouldn't fall off the platform which was elevated four feet. Good lift! That was my first time pulling over six hundred pounds. Team effort.

No one moves legit weight alone. No one gets there alone. You really want to bench press 500 lb. without someone spotting you? Nope. So, what do you do? Find a legit strength and conditioning coach that has a history of results. Then get your squad as close to as smart as the coach as possible. And hunt weaknesses. A Relentless approach to your training will propel you as an athlete. Get your training partners better, and then you have a squad to push each other.

Apply this concept to your key relationships in your life, then you've got it. If not, then we have more work to do.

Let's apply the training example to your position group on your team. You're the point guard in basketball. You're the starter, and there are two back-ups. You watch an extra hour of film daily; they are new and do not. Easy fix, right? Maybe. If you're weak-minded and insecure, you won't help them to develop winning habits. You'll continue to improve at a faster rate than them. So, you'll keep your starting position. And they won't do the extra work and won't progress at the same rate as you. You win the battle but lose the war. Why? First, you reinforced being weak-minded and being insecure. Second, you broke the Blocks of Being a Winner: Teamwork, Integrity, Kaizen, Enjoyment etc. Third, you ended up slowing your progress, and you did that intentionally. Fail! Why? How? If you watch extra film with your other point guards, here would be the natural results and progression:

- Your Teammates improve faster. When they get to play, they perform better. There is less of a drop-off when you leave the court. The team is better. Your team can win more.
- If you watch film with them and help, explain or point out different points of performance, then your act of teaching them will

further reinforce the knowledge for yourself. If you can teach the lesson, then you really know it.

- If you're competitive—and God, I hope so—then if they are watching an extra hour of film, you'll watch an extra two hours. And yup, now you're even better because you're pushed.
- When you make "deposits" to others (give of yourself and help them out), then you can ask for "withdrawals" later (things you receive). Don't just be a taker. Give first. Give often. It'll come back later.
- Did I mention a better chance of winning?! That's the idea, right?

Allies Versus Friends

You don't need that many friends, real friends. Probably a half dozen or less will suffice. You'll need many for different allies in different areas. Friends are those that are there to support, love, and care for you. It's what you would do for them. There is no limit to your or their love. It's given freely. And it's necessary.

Allies are those that lock arms with you to accomplish an endeavor. In this case, it's to get better at winning games. Now. Allies are required and critical for one main function: accountability. This person will hold you accountable and punish you for lack of effort and results. You will collaborate and discuss ideas. You will work together on new projects. It's a relationship where the goal is to accomplish a series of tasks and win. This is the person you want in your corner when you are training. He is the guy that says we aren't eating junk food; we aren't boozing up; we are going to bed early. And you must do the same for him. You may have different allies for different purposes, or one may serve in multiple roles. Or both. You'll need to figure it out. And you must adapt and evolve over time.

Maybe your dad was the one who got you a weight set and some books to get you started training. That's fantastic. It really is. It gets you started in the right direction. Eventually, though, you'll need a more advanced trainer to get you to the next level. Remember you will have to do more to squat 400 lb. than what you did to squat 300 lb. Most likely, your father will plateau as your coach. You will need a more advanced one. Still, be thankful that your father was a great ally here. Then it's time for the next one.

Tasks

- Find an ally for your training.
- Find an ally for your Nutrition and Recovery.
- Find a mentor ally to teach you the skills of the game. This could be a veteran on the team. It could be a retired athlete. You could have one of each. Be a sponge and soak up all the Knowledge. Fast! And then evolve it.
- Find a Teammate ally or two or three and join forces to improve beyond the normal practice schedule. Set the tone and culture for the team's standard. Culture will always be the team's number one asset.
- Find a Mindset ally that will get you mentally tougher and more focused.

Recent example: It was January of 2023. Ohio State lost in the semi-finals for the college football playoffs a few weeks ago. OSU's main receiver for the game was Marin Harrison Jr., the son of the Hall of Famer of the same name. Harrison Jr. took the jugs machine (the machine that spits out balls) with him to the hotel during the prep period before the game. He kept catching balls on his own time. I must believe he brought another receiver with him to practice. I bet he brought a defensive back who would harass him while catching balls. You see, these are allies. You're locked in together to attack and accomplish a task. Harrison played great in that game, too. Unfortunately, Georgia's team was better that day. It's a painful lesson: Even when you work your butt off, sometimes you still get beat. Winning does not care about you. Get yourself back up and fight again. And bring your Teammate along with you. You have a better shot then. And whatever amount of work the team has you do; it won't be enough for you to reach your fullest potential. Push. Move forward!

Impact and Influence

The late, great Jim Skerl, a 1974 graduate from St. Ignatius High School in Cleveland, Ohio, would say, "Actions speak louder than words. But words are never silent." Well, in fact, most everyone says the first part of that quote. But I never heard anyone say the second part. You can lead. You can inspire. You can get your Teammates to move forward. If you can, then you must. Why? Because you can! So do it. I shouldn't have to run you through the logic again of the benefits of improving your Teammates, so I won't. Just do it. The point is this: Do both. Lead primarily by your actions. But you also must have conversations with your Teammates to help lead them and be led by them. Both approaches are a must.

Tasks

- Broad task: Take your teammates in your position group through the Finding Your "Why" process that you went through earlier in this book. Ask them the same questions. Their "Whys" will be the reference point to remind them to move forward.
- Moderately specific task: Challenge them to do some Mindset challenges with you.
- Focused task: Teach them eight things they can do to help them sleep better.
- Pass on everything you know!

The All Blacks are the best. The New Zealand rugby team owns the highest winning percentage in the history of Earth's existence. The All Blacks state you should leave the jersey better than how you received it. James Kerr's *Legacy* highlights this approach beautifully. Your time playing your sport, for most (Remember the small fraction of a percentage that make it.), is an experience. It is not a career. To be clear, those who "make it" and go pro are the ones with the experience. Those who make it to the Statue level, that's the career. Someone wore your number before you. While you're wearing it, you represent that number and that team within the team's existence. You must honor those before you and carry it on. The game is bigger than you. Your team is bigger than you. Recognize that and do your best.

Pat Tillman was #42 at Arizona State University and #40 for the Arizona Cardinals. You think anyone else wears those numbers? Nope. Why? He left his pro career to serve his country as an Army Ranger in the war in Afghanistan, and he died while serving his country. Tillman was a monster on the field. He was overlooked and underestimated. Then he proved everyone wrong by wrecking offenses as a linebacker. But that wasn't enough. He gave football up completely early in his pro career to serve. He gave all he had for himself, his family, his unit, and his country. Be like the All Blacks. Be like Pat Tillman. Leave your jersey and leave this planet better than how you found it. That's impact.

CHAPTER 26

TEAMMATES - LEADERSHIP TEAM

You are the player. You've had multiple coaches to this point. Most likely there are multiple coaches on your team's staff currently. Obviously, your coaches are your Teammates too. Everyone is working toward the same goal of winning. Like it or not, finding the optimal ways to work together is critical.

Let's get the pervasive challenges out in the open:

- Not all Teammates have the same agenda. Some don't care so much about winning as they do about themselves personally.
- Not all Teammates act with champion Core Values: Integrity, Discipline, Kaizen, Teamwork, Enjoyment, and Sisu.
- Not all Teammates have the same work ethic.
- Not all Teammates are very competent. You will be amazed at those who get promoted prematurely and how it always comes crashing down.
- Teammates will have biases.

It happens with coaches. It happens in life. It happens in business. It happens in politics. It happens everywhere. It does not change the fact that the main job of the team is to win.

"The enemy of my enemy is my friend." – Sun Tzu, *The Art of War*

The main enemy for the team is losing. There are a multitude of other enemies within a team to note. But the sole, main enemy is losing. And there could be a scenario where you don't love your coach. He may not love you. But the coach's enemy is losing. Your enemy is losing. Therefore, your coach must be your friend to help you fight the enemy of losing. Then, you must find a way to get along and work together. You must work to respect and optimize your relationship. It is imperative you find a way to work together to win.

Yourself

Everything starts with you. Always and forever. Smash yourself, smother yourself, drown yourself with this question: What can I do first to lead myself and my team by my actions at the extreme highest level? "Actions speak louder than words, but words are never silent." So first, let your actions speak for you. Remember, culture is the team's number one asset. Your head coach and position coaches have a culture, and they are working to shape it into their vision. You must conduct your business supremely. Your job is to lead yourself and implement the coach's culture and vision.

Coaches

You don't know everything. Neither do your coaches. Hopefully they know more than you; they usually do. And guessing just makes things worse. So don't bother doing that either. Never mind that everyone is guessing and assuming all the time. How bad do coaches guess? About half of all first round QBs taken in the NFL draft end up being busts. That means teams of coaches, GMs, etc. work to select a player who ends up being a bust. Then Tom Brady was passed over by thirty-two teams of coaches five times before one team got it right in the sixth round. Geeze! What does this mean for you? Good question. Here's your process when dealing with coaches:

1. Be respectful while being real and authentic. Put yourself in their shoes and listen first. Learn. Be "all in" when dealing with them.

2. Your "eye test" will show up again here. Your attitude and body language are critical. If you're saying "yeah, yeah, blah, blah, blah" here. Think about when you ask a lady or man out. You read and observe their body language. You know if he or she is interested in you or not. So, yeah. . . it matters.

3. Always execute the coach's plan and vision as best you can. And work to get your teammates to do the same.

4. What level of athlete are you? Pretender? College Athlete? Pro? Or are you the Statue? Depending on which one you are, over-execute the plans and directives. Champions do more.

5. Be aware. The head coach is managing the assistants. Each assistant has a group he's trying to get to perform at the highest level. Often, he's speaking to the group. Not everyone in that group will be on the same athlete level. Be aware and understand that.

6. Remember, you are on your own path. Your path is to advance all the way to the end, whatever that end will be for you. Occasionally and consistently, you must ask the coach what else you can do. Must. Must. Must. Next level sub-process:

    a. Make an appointment.
    b. Type up an agenda with the questions dealing with your Inch Blocks. Bring one copy for you and one for the coach. Or even better, get it to him in advance so he can prepare as well. Also, it won't be a shock for him when you meet.
    c. What is the number one thing I can do to improve my Mindset?
    d. What is the number one thing I can do to improve my Knowledge and play in my sport and position?

e. What is the number one thing I can do to improve my interaction with the Teammates?

f. What is the number one thing I can do in my Training?

g. Ask if there is anything else you can improve.

h. Then you must over-execute here as well. Do this yourself and with anyone else. At the highest level of performance, the top 1 percent will be forced to drag the other 99 percent along with them to perform even higher. Just the way it is. Fact.

i. Set a deadline. Set a carrot and stick. Let your accountability ally know. Reevaluate weekly. And make another appointment to do it all over again. Win.

My son Sam executed this approach right after his high school junior season. I helped him go over everything and write out what he wanted to discuss with his coach. Sam did his SWOT analysis from his perspective. He wrote out his goals for senior season: Win his sectional and be named all-conference. He made an appointment with his coach and typed up two copies. His coach said it was the most well-prepared meeting he had ever had with a player. They discussed a number of things and then had a plan for next steps. It was smooth, easy, and impactful. It was a huge help.

Note: You will find an After Action Report (AAR) in the Process section of this book. This way you can have a process for assessing your games and your season with your coaches.

7. Use your brain! You are not a drone. Think. What else needs to occur on your end that you weren't told to do? What you were told as a team was the minimum. What the coach told you individually was the next level. That last Inch is what you can come up with on your own to do.

8. Move Forward. Relentlessly.

Other Leaders

There are other leaders and coaches on your team: athletic directors or general managers, bosses in the workplace, team captains, strength coaches. There are also leaders of the team's culture and attitude. Can you think of a situation where the above process isn't a great starting point? I can't. Then, as needed, repeat the process with the right person in that leadership group. As the starting pitcher on the team, how often do you really need to meet with the athletic director? Probably never. If you happen to bump into him or her at a team banquet or other dinner, could you simply ask for one piece of advice on how to improve as an athlete? Sure can. So, ask. Get more information and ideas. It can't hurt.

Personal example: I was elected president of my fraternity, Kappa Alpha Order, at Purdue University my senior year in college. My chapter was terrible at the time by most standards. We were downgraded to a "focus chapter." This meant that if we didn't improve in over forty areas over the next two years, then our chapter would shut down. Two things helped turn it around. First, I applied the accountability lessons and process I learned while running my job as the owner of the College Pro Painters franchise. I ran that business for three years in college to pay for my tuition. Second, I contacted the fraternity's prior presidents and influential alumni. I sent them letters asking for advice, processes, guidance, etc. Each person responded quickly. And it helped tremendously. It helped me create buy-in from the alumni. It also gave me concrete actions and tasks to follow. I didn't have to think about everything. Other great leaders had plenty of answers for me too.

Between using a weekly accountability model, I learned from running a business and the best ideas from prior leaders, I was able to map out a plan for the following year. One year later, at the end of my term, I was at our national convention in Atlanta. Thirty-eight of the assigned tasks were completed by then. Out of 113 chapters nationwide, we were recognized as a Most Improved Chapter. Win. There is help out there. Just ask. Write it down. And move forward.

CHAPTER 27

TEAMMATES - SUPPORT TEAM

No one gets there alone. It takes a village. Stop what you're doing right now and make a list of anyone that has sacrificed and helped you along the way. Go to the store and get thirty blank thank-you cards. Handwrite those people a message of gratitude and specifically thank them for what they've done for you. Put in there how you received help from their efforts, time, money, and guidance. You do owe some people right now. Be thankful. And communicate that you are thankful. Relentlessly.

There were people you needed to get you to where you are today. Some of those people will continue to help support you for years to come. And you will also pick up new people in your life who will help you and support you. Who? Family. Friends. Medical professionals. Jesus. Employees. Local people who cheered for you and bought your jersey. Professional colleagues. Financial advisors. Your priest or pastor. Nutrition and recovery coaches. The graduate assistants who clean your jersey. The administrative assistant helps to keep the coaches on target who help keep you on target to win next week. The list is endless.

Integrity: How you do anything is how you do everything.

Teamwork: The strength of the wolf is the pack. And the strength of the pack is the wolf.

Enjoyment: You must work your ass off Relentlessly. It's easier with a team you like to work with.

Let's be real. Some people suck sometimes. Some people suck all the time. And you can pick your friends, but you cannot pick your family. Your spouse or significant other will be critical to your Mindset. This person will help offload some of the domestic workload for you to work more on your craft. If you change teams at a high level, then your family will have to move with you or stay behind. Again, the list goes on and on. The point is this: Be thankful. Help them. And pass it on.

This won't take long. Just get out your journal, a notebook, your Inch Planner or App. During one of your reflective sessions, calm yourself and breathe. Think about everyone that has helped you along your journey. Then think about those that will be helping you today, tomorrow, and this year. Write down your list.

Why rank the support group? There is only so much time in the day. There are only so many resources. For some, your parents are 70 percent or more of your support group. For others it may be a local preacher or pastor at the religious center because your parents aren't in the picture. That's totally fine. And if you only have so much time and resources, then you must choose how you'll spend it.

Be real. Tell them what you're doing. You are on a path. You are going to play varsity basketball and graduate with a high school diploma. For some, that's a ton! I did great in high school academically. But in my sophomore year, I was cut from the only sport I played consistently growing up, basketball. No varsity letter for me. I had to learn an entirely new sport outside school for my athletic outlet, racquetball. Then I had to personally pay 90 percent of my way to compete in that sport. So, for some of your teammates, a degree in high school and a varsity letter is a big deal. And it really is. And that's great. Truly.

But again, be real with your supporters. Tell them the path you are on. Tell them your hopes and dreams. Let them know. It will help them. They will "buy in" to your hopes and dreams. They will receive satisfaction when the person they are helping succeeds. It further strengthens your Teamwork together.

Educate them. Hopes and dreams are nice, but utterly useless. Once you have a plan and are working on your plan, then your hopes and dreams can become powerful to the point of changing teams, cultures, and families. For example, let the cooks know that the care taken to provide healthy food and snacks makes up 60–70 percent of your physical success. Let your support team know that their efforts impact you in a real way. And thank them.

Thank them more times than you can count or remember. Everyone hates the entitled athlete. Don't be that jerk. Be the person who is gracious and appreciative. It's the right thing to do. It goes a very long way. And your support team will do even more for you in the end.

The Basics

- Keep everyone's birthday in your calendar. And say happy birthday. Or buy a ton of generic birthday cards and write them a note.
- Give them a Christmas or holiday card.
- Deliver a handwritten note.
- Call them or speak to them directly to thank them.
- Do something for them.
- At home, help your family and Teammates. Never be lazy. I've been around those types too. The amount of resentment that builds up is so great; no one ever wants to help the freeloader ever again.
- Tell others or tell their boss how one of your support Teammates has helped you specifically.

When you need something, be deliberate. Example: "Mom, I'll need rides to and from practice four days per week. Games are Saturday mornings over the next four months. I already talked with one of my teammates. He said his mom can help carpool. So now you'll only need to split half the rides. If we can get one or two more teammates' parents to help, then it will be even less work for you. I'm playing basketball so I can work to earn a college scholarship at best. At worst, I want to help our team win, earn a varsity letter, and make a difference at school."

Another example: Now you must win. And you must win for them. The offensive line in football is tasked with opening holes so the running back can "win" some yards and hopefully score. The line sacrifices and works to give the running back the opportunity to advance for the team. It's a selfless act and the only way the back can advance the ball forward.

It's the same with your parents. Driving you to practice does not help them. They sacrifice their time and resources for you to practice, play, and win. So do it! You know what travel sports costs? They cost families. Entire families will go to Florida for a three-day tournament. Vacations are put on hold. Tons of money is spent. Sometimes siblings who want nothing to do with the event are dragged along. And usually, any time spent in church is now gone too. And you might not even be that good! So, you better work your butt off and win for them. I truly believe what Tim Grover preaches. He says that if you're going to ask something of your family, then be specific. If you need three years to go out and give this sport a shot to go pro and start earning the money that changes a generation, then by God, do not take three years and a day. Get it done in under three years. Go all in and move forward.

And when it's all said and done, you have not even come close to thanking everyone enough. I know I haven't. No one has. And anyone who was especially hard on you and held you accountable, those are your true heroes. Accountability is not fun. The hard ally in your life was probably loving you the most. And you know it.

Who else is on your support team? Doctors and medical staff? Yes. Your financial planner? Yes. The recovery staff (e.g., masseuses, trainers, physical therapists)? Yes. Your agent? You betcha! Are there others? Darn right, there are. So now what? Well, some of them you must work with to advance. The team doctor is the team doctor. You'll need to work with him or her. What about other doctors? Yes. You'll need to have an Unbreakable Team at your disposal for you to function at the highest level. If you're on your path to excellence, can you have your babysitter late every day to watch your kids? Of course not. Everyone in your life matters. Act accordingly.

Results matter, right? Well, if they didn't, you wouldn't need this book. There is a reason there is a scoreboard. There have been athletes inside and outside my gym that have tweaked their knee. My wife tore her ACL once, and a second time, she tore her meniscus. What kills me is when athletes want to get their knee fixed but only look at the cheapest orthopedic doctor in their insurance network. They want to get their knee fixed, but they go to a guy that does knees, hips, ankles, shoulders, you name it. Not my wife. She went to Dr. Klootwyk. He only does knees. He's done knees for decades. He's the knee doctor for the Indianapolis Colts and Indiana State University's football team. He's the best in the Midwest, bar none. His entire staff is top notch. The staff is Relentlessly thorough. Scores of professional athletes have their pictures on his office walls, including my wife's picture. This dude is a legit stud. Go to him. The point is this: Up your game and surround yourself with the support staff you need. Hunt and interview your options and find the best one you can find. Get everyone on the same page and reward them accordingly. "It takes a village" is the phrase for raising a child. Well, it takes a village to produce an elite-level athlete.

The flip side is true too. If you live with a bunch of partying, drunk roommates, move out. If your financial guy doesn't have the answers or a support team himself, get a new guy. If your trainers don't have all the tools to help you heal, then you need to find outside trainers to fill in the gaps. If you have no clue on how to eat on your own, then you better absorb every word in our Nutrition section or hire a chef to make it happen for you. Here, the point is the opposite of the last point. "Hire someone" slowly when you're adding to your support team. But "fire quickly" once you know it's no longer a good fit. Hard example: I'll get into this more later in the Training section, but often in high school and college, you must do the team workouts. They're a must. And I get it. I understand why. On the flip side, everyone is fallible and makes mistakes. Definitely me included. If you're not progressing to becoming the best athletic specimen you can potentially become, you must hire an outside coach to fill in the gaps. The training gods over at WestSide Barbell in Columbus, Ohio have been doing it for decades. I've had to do it for my own kids and the athletes that come to my gym. I've seen it time and time again. Get the right people on your team because it still takes what it takes. Own your results and progress. Get others to help you too if your current group can't get the job done. And if I haven't said it enough, thank those on your support team more times than you can count!

Process

1. Take a moment and sit silently to think and reflect.
2. Make a list of those who help you. Make it as comprehensive as possible.
3. Rank them in order of workload and impact. The person who presses your suits and shirts once a month is great. The staff that makes and provides all your food at the training facility is greater. Both are amazing and critical. But one group provides more of an impact.
4. Be real. Be honest. Be transparent.

5. Thank them. Ask them how you could help them out with something.
6. Ask them for help.
7. Win for them and be "on time."
8. Pass it on.

CHAPTER 28

TEAMMATES - WAY OF INCHES

L et's work. Reminder here: For this test, focus solely on being a Teammate. That's it. The following is the Inches Way: Teammates section of the Assessment Test:

TEAMMATES

Players

- 10 Points: You are a captain of your team.
- 7 Points: You respect your Teammates, and they respect you. You work well with everyone and help get them better.
- 4 Points: You get your job done well and don't cause problems on your team. You mostly focus on yourself and not others.

POINTS: _____

Coaches

- 10 Points: You are the first one at the facility, last to leave, leader of your team, inform coaches, act as the "pulse of the team," are positive and upbeat, Relentless, and tough all the time.

- 8 Points: You mostly perform the duties listed above.
- 6 Points: You sometimes perform the duties listed above.
- 4 Points: You rarely perform the duties listed above.
- 0 Points: All else.

POINTS: _____

Professional Groups (teachers, trainers, medical staff, janitors, etc.)

- 10 Points: You are always respectful and professional, positive, supportive, and helpful.
- 8 points: You are mostly the qualities listed.
- 6 Points: You are sometimes the qualities listed.
- 4 Points: You are rarely the qualities listed.
- 0 Points: All else.

POINTS: _____

Kaizen

- 10 Points: You have a process for improving and adhere to it without fail.
- 8 Points: You mostly have a process and adhere to it.
- 5 Points: You occasionally have a process and adhere to it.
- 0 Points: All else.

POINTS: _____

Teammate Mentor

- 10 Points: You have one and connect weekly.
- 8 Points: You have one and connect monthly.

- 5 Points: You have one and connect quarterly.
- 0 Points: All else

POINTS: _____

How effectively are you working with a Teammate accountability ally (or allies)?

- 10 Points: You and your ally review your results weekly, enforce a "carrot/stick," and adjust.
- 7 Points: You and your ally review your results monthly and sometimes enforce "carrot/stick."
- 4 Points: You and your ally review your results quarterly.
- 0 Points: All else

POINTS: _____

You know your number one Teammate Strength (Competitive Advantage):

- 10 points. Otherwise: 0 points.

POINTS: _____

You know your number one Teammate Weakness (Weak Link):

- 10 points. Otherwise: 0 points.

POINTS: _____

You know your number one Teammate Opportunity (Target):

- 10 points. Otherwise: 0 points.

POINTS: _____

You know your number one Teammate Threat (Enemy):

- 10 points. Otherwise: 0 points.

POINTS: _____

TOTAL POINTS: _____
OVERALL AVERAGE (TOTAL POINTS /10) _____

You see your score. Retest yourself at the end of every quarter of the year (March 31, June 30, September 30, December 31).

Here we go again. Ask yourself a series of reflective questions and gauge your progress over the last quarter.

- Think about and write down your tribe of Teammates. These are the main people with whom you must work well to win. It's your position group, the leaders on your team, and your support group. Who's in your tribe?
- Does your tribe know you are a unit or need to be a unit? If not, meet with them face-to-face and tell them immediately what you're doing and your plans. James Clear: "If you want to be in the top 1 percent of a particular domain (your sport), then you can't take your cues from and follow the social norms of 99 percent of people. This is harder than it sounds. We are wired to imi-

tate. The further you want to climb, the more carefully you need to construct your tribe."

- Will you hold each other accountable? If not, then they are your friends, not allies. It's not the same. Your tribe must be allies too.
- Kaizen: Will you get your tribe 1 percent better? Will they get you 1 percent better? How? When?

SWOT Analysis

This time around, you must perform multiple SWOT analyses. The main analysis will be for your actual teammates. Then you will need to conduct an analysis for your leadership team as well as your support team. Don't sleep on this piece. Do it. Integrity is a Core Value.

- Strength:
  - List them all.
  - What are your top three?
  - What is your number one Strength (Competitive Advantage)?
- Weaknesses:
  - List them all.
  - What are your top three?
  - What is your number one Weakness (Weak Link)?
- Opportunities:
  - List them all.
  - What are your top three?
  - What is your number one Opportunity (Target)?
- Threats:
  - List them all.
  - What are your top three?
  - What is your number one Threat (Enemy)?

Teammates Way of Inches

Where must you be to win? This is with your teammates, leadership team, and support team. You can see your Advantages, Weak Link, Opportunities, and Enemy. Now list the actions that must occur. Must. Schedule the actions. Attack. Be Relentless. Then reevaluate.

Basic example: You play middle linebacker. Find the priority to attack. There are two middle (Mike) backers and two outside (one Sam and one Will) backers. Competitive Advantage: You and the other Mike are always on the same page, know the plays, are in the right position, and hit Relentlessly, no missed tackles. Weak Link: One of your Sam backers is consistently out of position. Opportunity: Have a "shut down" linebacking core that stops all runs, short passes, and passes over the middle. Threat: your team gets run on every play on the strong side and you get gashed for yards up and down the field and lose. Next steps: schedule extra film review with all linebackers three times/week for one hour each time. Quiz each other during the review. Then over-communicate when you're on the field. Miss review? Two hundred push-ups. Don't communicate? Two hundred push-ups. Reevaluate each Monday morning during the season. Let your position coach know what you're doing to get support from the leadership team. Let the film guys know what you need to get support from the support team. Move forward! Win!

10 Teammate Habits

No idea what to do next? Shoot, after that last example you should have at least one idea of what to do. Your mantra is Relentless. Apply it here. Remember, Statue > Pro Athlete > College Athlete > Pretender.

1. Lead by example in all things: weight room, attendance, attitude, etc.

2. Ask questions of your leadership team. Ask the right questions. Ask the hard questions. Example: you get five plays/game on special teams in football. Question: "Coach, what do I do to get fifty plays in a game?" Be painfully explicit. Use Grant Cardone's 10X Approach and get ten times more than what you're normally getting. Already on the field? "Coach, how can I dominate at a level that is ten times more than what I'm already doing?

3. Get your position group on the same page like in the example above. You play D in soccer, then you, the goalie, and the rest of the back guys need to have the same approach.

4. Take notes!

5. Find a mentor. Yesterday! Find multiple mentors if you can.

6. Get your home life, chores, and affairs in order. Keep your room and place clean and organized. By the time you're done with this book, you will have too much work to do and will screw it up if you are not organized at home.

7. Thank everyone that helps you more times than you can count.

8. Be Relentless in the weight room in training and getting your teammates stronger, faster, better. Watch them for mistakes and help them train better.

9. Read every day for twenty minutes on how to get better. Then tell your position group what you learned every Monday.

10. Own everything. Anything goes wrong? Claim it. Anything goes right? Thank and mention the team. Praise publicly. Criticize privately.

<u>Scan the following QR code</u> or visit: https://athlete-builder.com to access and download the assessment in this chapter and other resources (free nutrition resources and free workout programs).

CHAPTER 29

TRAINING

The Mindset Block is my favorite Block by far. Why? Your Mindset controls and dictates action. Your mind is everything because your actions make the impact and alter you and your environment. That is usually the goal. Following the natural progression here, the Training Block is my second favorite Block. This is where we work. The grind. The physicality of Training provides a real, meaningful test for your Mindset. Both Blocks are fully intertwined. You walk into a dark room (physical), you want (mind) to see better (physical). Then you turn on the light (physical). Your mind receives what it wants.

This is Training. It takes what it takes. You must do something physically to be rewarded (faster time, score a goal, block a goal attempt, make a shot, catch a ball, tackle someone, block someone, defend someone, kill someone). Your Training enables you to perform your desired task better. It satisfies your mind's requests. The more your Mindset pushes you, the more your Training advances.

Here is your "level up" approach. It's a Mindset thing. Look at your entire twenty-four-hour day as your training hall. Your Training is not limited to the weight room, your Knowledge in the film room with the coaches, the practice field, or the game itself. It's more. Your Training is impacted by everything around you: your environment, your tribe and Teammates, the Nutrition that enters you, and how you recover from training. Recognize that you must be more diligent in each Inch Block because each Block impacts the other Blocks. Now it's time to discuss your Training Block. It's time to get to work.

Let's start with the basics. If you use most any respected resource on building an athlete, it will have a Hierarchy Triangle like the one below. Any undergraduate or graduate program will have one. CrossFit has one. WestSide Barbell has one. CSCS has one. The Hierarchy Triangle is true in all sports, health and wellness, and simply fitness. It's universally utilized and respected because it is true and current.

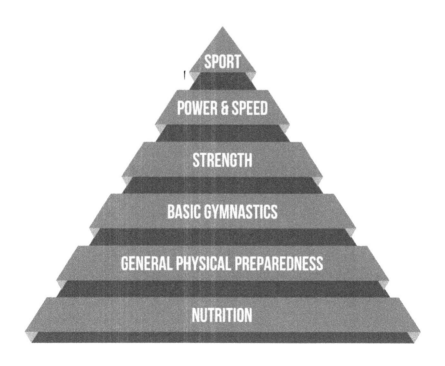

You must understand the underlying principles of the Hierarchy. Each position matters in size and scope. The order matters as well. The size matters. Everything matters. First, analyze the order:

Nutrition

Nutrition matters most because you cannot advance very far without it. "You can't outwork a bad diet." For example, lifting all day long without taking in protein will not advance you because your muscles need protein to grow. Also, taking in protein all day, or steroids for that matter, without training will not get you strong and fast. What you put into your body matters. The amount matters more and more as you add more physical demands. Most strength and conditioning coaches, trainers, body builders, runners, strongmen, CrossFitter, and powerlifters estimate that your Nutrition is between 60–75 percent of your success. I usually estimate it's about two-thirds, 66 percent. That's why the entire next Inch Block is about Nutrition.

GPP: General Physical Preparedness

Are you in shape or not? "Well, I don't need to be in shape to lift heavy!" Wrong! You might not need to be in much shape to squat or bench press 100 lb. It'll take more sets and reps in a normal training session to bring your numbers from 100 lb. to 200 lb. And the same is true to get to 300 lb. How many sets and reps will it take to get to a 600 lb. squat and 400 lb. bench press? These are standard numbers for most players in the NFL. The answer is it takes a lot more. Do you have 4 hours to spend daily in the gym? Remember this is on top of all the other training, not just two lifts. You'll have to add in the running, sprinting, etc. needed for your sport. The answer is that time and capacity are limiting factors. You must get more sets and reps in for you to grow and get stronger. You just don't have all day to do it. Therefore, you must be in some decent shape. You can only afford so long of a rest interval because you have more to do. And no one has 5-8 minutes between sets because of other obligations. You must be in shape to advance your Training. You must advance your Training if you're to advance in your sport.

General Gymnastics

This is not the gymnastics you see on T.V. during the Olympics. This simply means you need to move your body correctly. You must do this during your Training, at practice, during games, and with your posture when you walk, sit, and live your life. You need to learn the proper mechanics to throw a baseball or spike a volleyball. You ever see a hard-core wrestler play basketball? It's hysterical. They've never played. They always wrestle during basketball season. They don't have the mechanics down. It's a good time. You should watch. The point is that as you advance in the weight room, on the track or in your sport, you must learn all the levels and progressions for your body to move and recover optimally.

Strength

It's my favorite, and it's no secret. I love doing powerlifting and strongman work. In your sport, make no mistake. Strength cures a lot of sins! Everyone knows who the strongest kid on the team is. Everyone knows that as he gets better skilled his strength helps him dominate. Strength is critical in all sports in some form, even distance sports. Example: A power clean or a broad jump are both speed/power movements. Well, if you cannot deadlift 100 lb. (a strength movement), then you sure cannot power clean it. Who do you think jumps further? Someone that squats 100 lb. or someone that squats 500 lb.? Another example: A distance runner. Of course, their conditioning is critical. Their mechanics and stride are also critical. You ever notice when their stride shortens? A short stride makes them slower because they are not running optimally. Usually, it's their posture weakening because their core and back aren't strong enough to hold the optimal running pose during the race. This creates more work for the body which tires it out. Speed diminishes then. Lesson: get strong as possible and then apply it to the next spot on the pyramid to really dominate.

Speed and Power

If strength cures a lot of sins, speed and power kill. Like strength, everyone knows who the fastest and most powerful kid is on the team. You can really create some separation here between athletes as this puzzle starts to unfold. You have the best shot if you're consistently the first one to the ball or the first one to the spot on the field or the court to make a play. Getting their first is an enormous advantage. Speed and power are absolutely critical.

Sport

There are too many nuances in every sport to list. The ten-thousand-hour rule applies here. Being an expert here can put you on the path to the Statue. Learn every habit and trick of the trade that you can. Greatness requires it. The point of all the Training is for the athlete to apply his skills at his sport the best he can. Applying your skill is what matters most. Training just helps that.

Side note. The current generation of travel leagues and teams have real challenges for their athletes because of the year-round practicing. Most travel teams take the fitness and training "laws" and turn the pyramid upside down. They make the travel sport the base of the pyramid. Then it's speed work, like poorly programmed agility ladders. Strength and building a base of proper movement (basic gymnastics) for the body are never prioritized. Nutrition starts at home. So, we can't blame the coaches here. Result: repetitive use injuries have skyrocketed. Shoulders and elbows are wrecked for baseball/softball kids. ACLs are torn for soccer, basketball, volleyball, and others. It's really hard on the athletes. This is why we have to make some adjustments and fix it now.

In my generation, the kid lucky enough to play travel all-stars ended up being the best. Why? He received more reps in his sport than the other kids. No one else did. That was the separator. Today it's the norm. Everyone plays travel ball. But no one has "time" to get stronger and faster. Being the strongest and fastest kid is now the new separator because no one does it. Process change: take two to three days per week and get your kid into a legit gym with legit coaches. If he's strong, then he has a better shot of being safe from injury. Then he has a base to get faster and more powerful. Then look out!

Specializing early is a mistake. At best, it's simply not optimal. Why? Answer: The brain. Let's oversimply things here medically. If you repeatedly do something (math problems, sewing, fishing, cooking, playing basketball), your brain evolves and gets better at what you're doing. The neuro pathways become stronger and more effective. If you only do your "one thing", then your brain essentially gets into a rut and continues to groove its patterns. When you add another activity, the brain must groove in different pathways. It will learn new things and methods. It will advance again, but in a different way. Invariably, overlap and improvements will occur from one activity to another. Example: wrestlers are excellent at using their hands to create leverage against their opponents. It will also help them when they use their hands to block or tackle in football.

That's the science behind not specializing. In addition, playing another sport enables the athletes to "miss" his main sport. He won't be burned out then. He'll return to it rejuvenated and excited. "Well, what about just training instead of playing a second or third sport?" Answer: Kids should lift and train as soon as they can. But they don't need to do it four to five times a week, especially at an early age. They can play a second sport and get to the gym two or three times a week. (That doesn't mean playing two sports at one plus training. That's not sustainable.) Playing on another team helps him learn and develop the necessary skills to be a Teammate. Keep him in multiple sports throughout the year.

Bottom line: Like the laws of physics and nature, stick to the pyramid. There are no special snowflakes. The fundamentals are called fundamentals for a reason. Stick to those and over execute.

There are two more things to note and explain. First, initial improvement in any undeveloped segment is rapid and significant. Second, once a segment is maximized, the supporting segments must be improved more before the desired segment is advanced. Likewise, once your entire pyramid is optimized, the only way to advance is by increasing the size of the pyramid. This means all sections of the pyramid: Eat more food to enable strength gains; address your mobility to perfect movement patterns; get stronger, faster, and more powerful; and apply it to your sport.

The first point should be obvious. If you've never touched a barbell in your life, then the first six to twelve months you use it should be nothing but fun. You know absolutely nothing in the beginning. Therefore, every training session should result in some new PR (Personal Record). Your technique will improve rapidly. You'll get stronger quickly. Simply learning the basics will provide quick gains each week. Then after twelve to twenty-four months, reality will set in. Your main lifts won't improve 20 lb./month any longer. You learn it takes work to progress. That's okay. Becoming better is a great time! So, enjoy it.

Like never touching a barbell, never doing anything to impact a level of the pyramid means you're at the bottom of the learning curve. That's fine too. Your gains for the next twelve to twenty-four months will be easy and fun. So, enjoy the ride.

Speed and power: You haven't done anything to get faster up until this point. If you spend the next six months working on it, gains will be significant and rapid. It's not that speed is the key. It's not that a speed coach is the key. It's that you've never done anything before to work on speed, and now you have. Of course, you'll get better immediately. Then the inevitable plateau hits. You've been power cleaning 155 lb. and you want to get to 185 lb. The problem is that you can only deadlift and front squat 185 lb. That's the problem. You must back track and build up your strength numbers first. Why? The strength segment supports the power/speed segment. Build your deadlift and front squat to 275 lb., and you'll see that power cleaning 185 lb. is easier. Think I'm crazy? You ever watch the top strongmen in the world power clean weight? It is one of the ugliest things you'll ever see. Brian Shaw will slowly stand up and essentially reverse curl 335 lb. like it's nothing. There's no hip pop to shoot the weight up. There is no discernable Olympic movement technique. It's terrible. So how then? Well, he deadlifts over a thousand pounds! That segment of his triangle is enormous. So of course, he can power clean that weight. It's only a third of his deadlift max.

Louie Simmons always said that "a pyramid is only as large as its base." It's in reference to the triangle concept. Once you advance past the initial learning curve gains, you must work more to improve. Whatever it took for you to have a 36″ vertical jump or run a 4.80 forty-yard time will not work for you to improve. You must do more. Your pyramid must get bigger in all components. You must have better Nutrition. You must move even better with better technique. You must get stronger, faster, and more powerful. You must learn more nuances in your sport. Everything matters. Improvement takes more. Grow your pyramid. Relentlessly.

CHAPTER 30

TRAINING - LET'S GET AFTER IT

Where do we begin? Volumes, manuals, and textbooks are dedicated to this topic. Entire courses will spend semesters on this topic. How can we begin to tackle the subject here? This is not an all-encompassing training manual. Instead, I will lay out the basics and directives for you to improve. KISS. Keep It Simple Stupid. I take the basic laws of nature of physics and apply them. Relentlessly. It forms a creed and framework. Then it's easy to move forward. Don't break the laws. Let them guide you to success. It's just like our Core Values.

You don't know what you don't know. Find a coach. It's a must. You can get books, and they can be adequate. But find a coach. Train with a group. I asked my father once what should I do to get stronger and better to play high school basketball? He had two answers: First, just do a lot of pushups. Second, shoot a lot of shots. That was it. Nothing more. I could get behind shooting a lot of shots to develop the basketball skills. But the only thing for my body was pushups? That's it? He was an idiot at health and fitness. He died young and was unhealthy his entire life. In fact, he never saw my gym. Lesson: don't listen to stupid people in the area you want to improve in. Find a coach. And find a legit, good one.

Let's assume you can't find a coach and you must do it yourself. Then go with the basics. Jim Wendler's *5/3/1* book is excellent for the basics on getting stronger. Or go to Dave Tate's site; www.elitefts.com for all the articles. There is amazing content there. One of the gold standards is anything put out by WestSide Barbell (www.westside-barbell.com). Tate came from WestSide Barbell. But find a resource or coach. Do not be dumb, driven cattle. When you talk to a coach ask their philosophy on Training? Interview them. And then learn everything you can.

GPP

This book is designed for athletes preparing to play at a high level: varsity high school, college, and pro athletes as you progress. If you're younger, middle-school age, then do the following: Find a coach! Get off your phone and get outside. Run and jump, pushups and pull-ups, lunges, and plank holds. Be as active as possible.

Now for high school, most likely there is a strength and conditioning coach at your school. Perhaps you must take a class, typically called APC, Advanced Physical Conditioning. This could be a good start. Sometimes it is. Other times some schools don't even have a program for strength and conditioning. Funding isn't always a priority here. Either way, we must evolve and improve.

If you're still not sure what to do, then follow the pyramid. We'll discuss Nutrition in a different section of the book. For Training, start by getting in a basic level of shape. Do some rudimentary conditioning. When doing conditioning, think about your sport. Example: playing baseball does not require 5-mile runs. But doing twenty to twenty-five minutes of interval training (30 seconds of work and thirty seconds of rest) would be beneficial. Or doing moderate sprint workouts (sprint at 75 percent for ten seconds and fifty seconds to walk back). Remember, this is conditioning, not speed work. You want to build your basic capacity so you can have the stamina required to handle the higher levels of training later in the day (weightlifting, calisthenics, core work, speed, and power work, and then the sport-specific work). Then test and see. Example: If you're in shape enough to get through the weightlifting but start to fade during the speed work, then you'll need to increase your

GPP base, or your stamina/endurance. Conversely, if at the end of each day's training you don't feel overly fatigued, then your GPP level is adequate. You're doing just fine. You can allocate more of your time and energy to the levels above on your pyramid.

For building your capacity and GPP, interval training provides the most bang for your buck. Getting your heart rate up and down and up again will get you in shape quickly. And most likely, your sport operates in intervals of hard work and resting or lighter work. At the initial stage of your training a basic interval of thirty seconds of work followed by thirty seconds of rest is great. Or forty-five seconds of work followed by fifteen seconds of rest. Later in your career, it could be different: ten seconds of a hard sprint and thirty seconds of a moderate jog. You'll tailor your interval training to your sport's demands.

Gymnastics, a.k.a. Moving Correctly. Hunt Weaknesses.

There is more to running quickly than simply leaning forward and moving your feet. The same is true for lifting. The technique required to clean and press 315 lb. is much more than doing the same with just the bar. To be clear, the technique is the same. The repercussions for poor technique are more severe when lifting 315 lb. versus an empty 45 lb. bar. As an athlete, you must be proficient in a multitude of movements. When a coach or a game applies stress, then movement patterns will be challenged. This is great. It's exactly what we want. You won't "rise to the occasion." You'll default to your level of training. So, if you want to clean and press 315 lb., then you'd better learn the best technique to do that.

You will have sport-specific technique too. If you want to throw a 90-mph fastball, you'll constantly work on your throwing mechanics. Whether you're cleaning weight or throwing a ball, make sure someone is watching. You cannot see where your form breaks down, but your coaches or teammates can. Tell them to watch for breaks in your technique. Then you can learn and get better. It's critical. I remember when a newbie in my gym said, "It sure must be nice to be able to squat so much and not need anyone to coach you and tell you what you're doing wrong." I laughed out loud. It was the opposite of what's true. It was one of my best squat sessions that day. I had 425 lb. on the bar and 150 lb. of chains added to the bar. The guy was watching and quickly learned he was wrong. I had three spotters and two coaches watching. One coach was giving me cues ("Hips back, drive into the bar, squeeze your butt!") throughout the lift. The other coach was watching to see what parts of my body and lift struggled most. He also watched for what components were slower, indicating relative weakness. Did my chest cave in? Knees cave in? Stall at a sticking point? The point is this: At all levels you must hunt your weaknesses. Constantly be diligent in improving your form and technique. If you know the parts of the body that are weaker relative to other parts, then you can select the corresponding accessories to strengthen the weaker areas. Then you get better faster. Process is king.

The above example is only for one lift in the weight room. There are plenty more. And then you must improve your form and technique to play your sport better. It will take a million shots or more in basketball to be at the Statue level. (Kobe was doing five hundred "makes," not "shots," from each corner and the top of the key at breakfast, lunch, and dinner. For years! That's just those three spots.)

Strength

Remember, everyone knows who's the strongest on the team. Everyone knows that the strongest athletes have a lot of potential when they receive the ball or puck, or swing the bat. Strength is the main tool that allows you to build and optimize the next main tools: speed and power. It also protects and provides self-made body armor against impact and injury. Building strength requires building your Mindset. It takes real courage to stand or lay under a 600 lb. bar. Risk can be high. Your mind is your only shot of getting through the lift. I cannot stress it enough: Get as strong as possible mentally and physically. Now.

Basic Formulas, Rules, and Definitions

- Force is a function of an object and how it builds up Velocity. Force = Mass × Acceleration
  - Example: A 250 lb. linebacker picking up speed hits a 200 lb. running back who is running at the same speed. Who wins? The linebacker wins. Why? More force. Applied rule: The harder you hit someone, the less you feel it. Don't believe me? Here are two examples you can try:
    - Take two balls (like pool balls or golf balls) that are the exact same. Roll one slowly. Roll the other much quicker into the slow ball. What happens? The slow ball absorbs the impact mostly and bounces off the fast ball backward. The faster ball hits the slow ball and slows down but keeps moving forward.
    - Take two different balls (a pool ball versus a golf ball). Roll them at the same speed at each other. What happens? The larger ball hits the smaller ball knocking it backward. Same deal here.
- Work is a Force applied over a distance. Work = Force × Displacement
  - It's more work for me to move a wheelbarrow full of wood a hundred yards than to move an empty wheelbarrow the same distance. Why? Force is a component of mass. The heavier one has more mass and therefore more Work. The same is true if I run with it versus walking. Why? I'm accelerating more. Therefore, Work increases. It's also more Work to move it a hundred yards versus ten yards. Why? More distance.

- Velocity is the Distance traveled over Time. Velocity = Displacement / Time
  - What's your "forty time"? Your time in the forty-yard dash? It's traveling forty yards in so many seconds. You can convert that to a speed, or Velocity.
  - Running forty yards in five seconds equates to 16.36 mph. Running the same distance in four seconds equates to running 20.45 mph.
- Power is the Work done over a period of Time. Power = Work / Time. It is also a function of Velocity. Power = Force × Velocity.
  - Deadlifting 225 lb. requires you to stand up with the weight. Power cleaning 225 lb. requires you to stand up with the weight and pop it up into your front rack position. It clearly requires more Power. Why? It's a further distance traveled. The bar must also move quicker. It's a function of Velocity.

Why does this matter? Getting stronger requires more Force production. Move more mass, and Force increases. Strength training does this. Why does that matter? Increased Force allows you to exert more Force into the ground. This ability improves your Work. It improves your Velocity. It improves your Power. Why does that matter? Usually, the first one to the ball or spot on the field or spot on the court or fastest or most powerful has the best chance to win the battle in that moment. That impacts the game. That impacts winning and losing. And the reason to play the game is to win it.

Basics For Building Strength

Build absolute strength. This requires you to move a heavier and heavier weight over the same distance. The back squat is a basic example. More strength is required to squat 495 lb. versus 135 lb. Continue to build absolute strength in your main lifts and accessory lifts. You must be stronger than before to be able to do this.

Build speed strength. The label can be confusing. Essentially it means to move the same weight faster than before. If you're moving the same Mass at a higher Acceleration, then your Force production increases. To get very technical, moving a weight anywhere from 0.75 m/s to 1.0 m/s is an excellent target range. Today, more and more coaches and gyms use Velocity Based Training (VBT). They understand and value the need to move weight faster. There is a great connection between building absolute strength and building speed strength. Each impacts the other positively. Building absolute strength will help you move lighter loads faster. Also building more speed strength enables you to move heavier and heavier loads. The following are two critical points that provide enormous separators for athletes.

For each movement and set, move every rep (on the way up, not down) as fast as you possibly can. Every time. Even the warm-up sets. Every rep! Why? It creates more Force production. That's the point. More Force. The habit also prepares your nervous system for what's coming next, more weight. Most athletes are casual and undisciplined in their lighter sets. You must be Relentless. Disciplined. Push each set and rep. Make them count.

Most strength coaches only focus on the speed sets. When that's true, they truly fail their teams and organizations. It's really a shame when this occurs. Some coaches refuse to push up the absolute strength numbers. They are afraid. Fear cripples them because they worry about injury to the point of avoiding heavier weights. And those athletes are brutally underprepared. Their potential is critically diminished. And in their sport, they are at a significant disadvantage. Yes, their performance is less than it could be. But also, injury risk increases because others are more powerful. And in a game of force, no one wants to be the weaker athlete.

Example: Carson Steele was a great running back out of high school and ended up at Ball State University in 2021. He had very good speed.

He wasn't quite as shifty on a relative basis. His great "thing" was that he hit his holes and broke tackles. Every time. It also helped that he squatted 600 lb., benched 400 lb., and cleaned 315 lb. before age twenty. The thing was that he had close to those numbers prior to arriving at Ball State. His strength was a tool that fostered his speed and power. It enabled him to exert more force when he ran. It's a big reason why he would win the one-on-one battles. He ended up outgrowing the program and transferred to UCLA to start his third year.

Build repetition strength. Hypertrophy method. This requires more and more reps. Large sets of reps (between twelve and twenty) help you build more muscle. The lighter reps in a set don't build strength. That comes from fewer reps (five or fewer) that are much heavier. However, building more muscle enables you to increase your strength eventually. It still ties in.

Question: Which should you do (heavy reps, speed reps, or many hypertrophy reps)? Answer: Do all three. Apply each method to help you build your body for your sport. Keep building up your main lifts until you get to the point where you are in the top 10 percent for your position in your sport at an elite level. That's the target. Get to the Statue level. Also move the weights AFAP (As Fast as Possible). Velocity is built here. Lastly, when you do your accessories, at a certain weight, go AMAP (As Many as Possible). Say you're doing triceps push downs to build your triceps and arms. The weight is 40 lb., and the rep scheme calls for four sets of twelve reps. Well, you desire the most growth and muscle adaptation. This occurs when the muscle must strain severely to execute the task. This happens in the last one to three reps in the set. It only occurs when those reps are hard and meaningful. If you've done your twelve reps and you can do eight more, then keep going! Make it meaningful. Note: Do not fail at your reps. Leave one or two in the tank. Failed reps have a much higher correlation with injury. So go hard, but don't fail. It's the last one to three reps you can do that are hard with one or two reps left in the tank. That's the target.

Next, you make most of your money with your accessories. This should account for 80 percent of your day's training. The main lifts should account for 20 percent at most. Build the smaller muscle groups and it will tie into the overall, larger muscle groups. Then your main lifts will go up. Don't get me wrong, the 20 percent of the training with the main lift is necessary too. You'll move your main lifts up as well from that 20 percent. The point is not to be casual and, God forbid, comfortable in your training with your accessories.

Accessories process. Example: You have 4×12 triceps extensions as an accessory on an upper body day for the next four weeks. Week 1 looks like this:

- Twelve reps at 40 lb., thirteen reps at 40 lb., thirteen reps at 40 lb., twelve reps at 40 lb. (total of fifty reps at 40 lb.)

Week 2 must be better. Kaizen is a Core Value. You must get fifty-one reps or more at a weight of 40 lb. or more. Let's say you did this as an example:

- 40 lb. had the following reps for four sets: 13, 14, 14, 14. Good. You win. Fifty-five reps.
- Week 3 had all sets at fifteen reps. Sixty reps total. Perfect. Another win.
- Week 4, you go to 45 lb. and get the following: 12, 11, 11, 11 reps. Perfect. You're close to the twelve-rep targets and your weight went up over the four weeks. That's exactly what we want. That's the approach. That's the Kaizen Mindset. Attack in Training.

Strong Back = Strong Everything.

This is not a hard and fast rule or one you'll find in textbooks. It's a Jim Beebe rule. Why? Most athletes and coaches work extensively on the muscles on the front of the body (the anterior). The backside (posterior) gets neglected. What happens then? The same thing that happens whenever there is an imbalance: Injury risk increases dramatically. Look at the "running sports" basketball, soccer, even volleyball to an extent. The sprinting is very "quad-dominant," meaning the athletes' quadriceps get developed much more than their backside (glutes and hamstrings). What's the byproduct? ACL tears.

Look at throwers, pitchers, and baseball/softball players in general. Their upper backs and scapulae are critical in stopping their arms from throwing a ball. What happens when they are underdeveloped and weak? Elbow issues. Shoulder tears. Rotator cuff tears. Their arms, upper backs, and scapulae are not strong enough to hold everything together. Strength is critical. The travel teams are faced with a real challenge here. Their seasons are ten months or longer. They'll have multiple practices each week and five to eight games at the end of the week. The excessive demands on the athlete can lead to more frequent injuries. If they did some weight training three times a week, they could build the athlete to handle the wear and tear of the sport. And then the whole team would dominate.

I'm forty-eight years old. It used to be that in my day, in the late '80s and early '90s, that the kid who played travel ball would win. He'd play in high school and eventually college too. That was the separator. Why? Well, very few played travel ball. He got a lot more reps than everyone else. His sport IQ and skill were much higher. Now, today that's not the case. Everyone plays travel ball. It is no longer the separator. The playing field is level with the number of reps. But how many strength train? How many do it well? Some might do some work in the offseason for two months. Are people really that ignorant that they think it will last and help them the next ten months? It's ridiculous. The answer is the same as always: It takes what it takes. Either make time for strength training or make time for injury recovery. Strength training is now currently the main separator. The athlete will create his own competitive advantage. This could be a specific avenue to help the athlete win, especially if most others aren't doing it!

Take some further examples: If you can bench press 275 lb. and can only barbell row 135 lb., there's a problem. The ratios are off. You can press way more than you can pull in this instance. Those numbers should be closer together. Fix that. Add in more pulling: rows, pull- or chin-ups, face pulls, etc. Build that back up. Fix the imbalance so you're safer and better.

You can back squat 315 lb. and your front squat is 295 lb. That's way too close. Your quads are much stronger by comparison in this instance. Start squatting wider and keep the weight on your back. Build your glutes and hamstrings. Add in more leg curls and glute bridges. Fix the imbalance. These are two basic examples of imbalances. You and your coach must look for them and address them with your training. It's really a matter of problem-solving all the time. Keep adjusting your course of action Relentlessly.

Speed and Power

Strength is a huge tool. Now let's utilize it and build more speed and power. This really impacts athletic performance. There are four methods we employ mostly for this endeavor: jumps, landing jumps, sprints, and Olympic lifts. Before we explore those areas, note one thing: Remember to move yourself and your resistance training (weight training) as fast as possible. Always. For example, lighter weight squats (40–70 percent) must be performed AFAP. It's another form of speed training. The same is true for all lifts. This is critical.

Another principle: All methods work, and none of them work. And nothing works forever. It depends. A broad jump can be great. You're using your body weight for resistance. You can measure and track progress. It builds the fast-twitch type-II muscle fibers. It's awesome. Where is it *not* great? If executed incorrectly, it limits the benefits. If your knees cave in because your back side is weak, this is only great if you address and fix the weakness. It's terrible if you can't recognize it or simply do not improve it. It's also not great if it's the only jump you do. And in your sport how often do you ever jump, under control, forward, with two feet, and land with two feet while sticking the landing? It's rare. Do you understand why with everything, it depends?

So now what? Work on your broad jump for four to six weeks or until it stalls improving. Then change up the stimulus. Pick a different jump. Pick a single leg jump and repeat the process. Be sure to develop both legs of course. Then you can do rolling jumps where you perform four to six jumps in a row with the minimum amount of time spent on the floor between jumps (less than one second). Once this stalls, then mix in lateral jumps to each side or multiple jumps in a row on one leg, changing direction within each sequence. It's a lot more often that an athlete will push his bodyweight primarily with one foot in the direction of play on the field. Then it behooves us to practice and improve the same movement pattern.

One of the ways to improve your ability to apply force is to improve how you receive force. The basic example is to jump off something and land. Landing off a jump from a twelve-inch box isn't very challenging. It's more challenging landing on one foot. It's increasingly challenging when it's performed at higher heights and/or with more weight. When would this be important? Basketball players jump and land constantly throughout a game. Wide receivers and defensive backs jump and land all the time during a football game. You must prepare your body for impact. Adding in a few series of depth jumps (jumping off something) will help prepare the body for the impact of landing. It also prepares the body to receive force. If the body can receive force, then it's better equipped to apply force.

Short sprints are fantastic for developing speed and power. This can be performed several ways:

- Start in a comfortable "ready stance."
- Start in "blocks" like in track events.
- Start lying down on your belly. Or turn over and start from your back. This will simulate getting knocked down and having to jump up and run to the next play.
- Start shuffling to one side laterally and then turn and sprint twenty yards.
- Sprint up a hill. This is excellent for learning running techniques because it's hard to "hide" bad form when running up a hill.
- Sprint with resistance, like dragging a sled.

A few things to note, give yourself 90–100 percent of a full recovery between sprints. Sprinting "all out" is very taxing. Doing it while fatigued hinders your ability to sprint "all out." And Intensity = Results. You must be intense and sprint "all out" to achieve the desired results. You'll only need to perform sprints twice each week, but it will be helpful.

Olympic lifts (cleans, snatches, and jerks) are also useful in developing speed and power. Like any jumping motion, the body performs its "triple extension" when performing the Olympic lifts. Triple extension also occurs when you jump. A triple extension occurs when you fully extend your ankle joints, your knee joints, and your hip joints (jump). All three occur fully when you maximize your triple extension. With jumps, it's usually only your body weight. (You could wear a weight vest.) With the lifts, you are moving a barbell or dumbbell. The added weight is clearly more resistance and a very effective way of increasing your speed and power output.

What about developing speed and power for your upper body? Is it important to be powerful and explosive here? Absolutely it is. Jerks and push presses help a lot with upper body power training. Any form of throw will help as well. Med balls are great tools for catching and absorbing force. Med balls are also excellent for throwing, generating force. Any plyometric presses work well too, like plyometric pushups. I've also had athletes perform plyometric pull-ups. They would perform a pull-up so powerfully, they would propel themselves high enough to catch another bar over the first bar. They'd catch the second bar and control themselves back down to the first and then to the floor. Then it's time to repeat the exercise.

Here is what's great: Developing your speed and power will help you increase your absolute strength. The opposite is also true. Increasing your absolute strength will help you increase your speed and power. So, in which area do you spend your time? Both.

Putting It Together

First, let's assume you are not training with your school or with a coach/gym. If that's the case, then let's put out a basic template for training. You'll do one lower body day that is heavy. Then you'll do an upper body day that is light and fast. Third will be a lower body day that is light and fast. Last will be an upper body day that is heavy. This will span one week.

Warm-up

Start your session by getting your blood flowing with a light jog, by rowing on an erg machine or jumping rope, or other light exercise. Then get into a dynamic warm up with your upper or lower body depending on the day's training plan. Work in range of motion (ROM) drills, mobility, and box breathing for your body to move optimally. Start broadly with full-body movements. Then taper that down to more specific body parts, muscle groups depending on the day. Always warm up your core and back regardless of the day. Finish with exercise-specific movements.

Explosive Work

Jumps, plyometrics, Olympic lifts, throws, or catches should be done first prior to any strength training. For lower body days, spend fifteen to eighteen minutes on two to three exercises. Perhaps start with five sets of five jumps over hurdles. Then perform five sets of five jumps over five lower hurdles while on one leg. Then do the other leg. Last work on eight sets of two reps of hang cleans.

Strength Work

There are many ways to train consistently and systematically. I gravitate toward Louie Simmons's Conjugate Method approach at WestSide Barbell. Our gym has trained this way for years with consistent results. It is very effective and sustainable. It's not flashy and can be boring. But greatness comes from doing the fundamentals better than anyone else. Stick with the conjugate approach.

Max Effort Lower Day

Pick four main movements for your lower body: box squat, trap bar deadlift, front squat, and sumo deadlift. The first week, work up to a heavy box squat for about five reps. Then do two more sets (2×5) and 80–90 percent of the heaviest set you did that day. Next week, work up to a 5RM (five-rep max) trap bar deadlift. Again, perform two more back down sets (2×5) with the same number of reps between 80–90 percent. Week 3 is the same reps and process for the front squat. Week 4, it's the same reps and process for sumo deadlift. That's an entire month.

Next month, each max effort day, you will work up to a 3RM (three-rep max). It's back on box squat for Week 1 in Month 2. For example, work up to a heavy set of five reps in Month 1. In Month 2, work up to a heavy set of three reps. Then do your back down sets of 2×3 and 80–90 percent of the day's heaviest amount lifted successfully. Week 2 in Month 2 is trap bar deadlift for three reps and the back down sets. Week 3 in Month 3 is the same process for front squat. And it's sumo deadlift in Week 4 of Month 2.

Month 3, repeat the process but this time with a heavy one rep max. The back-down sets are a little different. Do 3×1 at 80-90 percent. Continue to rotate the exercises in Month 3 like the prior months. Month 4, repeat Month 1. Now you're set for your main lift on the Max Effort Lower Days.

Remember this is about 20 percent of the day's total training. The other 80 percent includes your explosive work in the beginning plus your accessories. For your accessories, pick three to five movements that build up your weaknesses for that day. Do reps schemes of six to twenty reps depending on the desired effect. A lower-body day should have some glute and hamstring work, some quad work, some back work, and always core work. Do core work as much as possible. It'll recover quickly. Pick a movement—glute bridges, for example—and do the same set and rep scheme over a month. You must try to improve the number of reps or weight for that exercise over the month. This is where you make your growth. You must smash your accessories to move your main lifts. Note: For any lower body work, a reverse hyper is gold for improving and healing. Find one or buy one and use it as much as possible.

For your core work, movements that keep your trunk stationary statically and/or while moving your extremities is optimal. Doing sit-ups has some benefits. But putting your spine in flexion/extension repeatedly is not great. If you're going to do that, then stick with standing abs with a band on pull-up bar. Stick with planks, weighted planks, unbalanced planks, Paloff press, and standing unbalanced static holds.

Finishers: If a body part needs a lot of blood flow for growth or healing, then pick a very light weight movement and do sets of fifty to one hundred reps.

Max Effort Upper Day

This is done exactly like the ME Lower Day. Pick four upper-body movements: bench press, shoulder press/military press, floor press, and close grip incline press. Month 1 will have sets of five reps. Work up to the day's max. Do your drop-down sets (2×5 at 80-90 percent of day's max). And rotate the next week. Month 2 will have sets of three and the drop-down sets. Month 3 will have sets of one rep. Month 4 repeats Month 1.

Again, pick your Accessories and try to PR each week. Pick three to four and address your weaknesses. Add in back work and core work. Then you'll be set. A few items to note: For the two lower body days my back work usually consists of vertical pulls (pull-ups, chin-ups, lat pull-downs, etc.). The upper body days have more horizontal pulls (ring rows, single-arm rows, barbell rows, etc.). I change my core work each day. So, one day would be upper core, like from rollouts. The next day would be my sides, obliques from side plank holds, static holds, etc. The third day would be lower core: flutter kicks, leg raises, dead bugs, etc. The fourth day would be a static hold: plank hold, or a variation of it.

Dynamic Effort Lower Day

Pick one main lower movement for that month. Box squatting is excellent for athletes. So let's start here and remain here for a while. You'll want to get between twenty to thirty reps, ideally around twenty-four reps. Rep schemes of 8×3, 12×2, 5×5 are great. Week 1, do all sets at 60 percent. Week 2 is 65 percent. Week 3 is 70 percent. Week 4 is 75 percent. The next week, start the process over and repeat. We won't get into accommodating resistance (bands and chains) in this book. You should really have a coach if you've progressed to this level. But keep the sets and reps in this range and you'll be solid.

You'll need more, different accessories for this day as well. Continue to build up your lower body and posterior with these. Do more sets and reps on your accessories on your dynamic days. Your max days are more taxing because of the higher loads. Consequently, you can handle more volume on your dynamic days. Still hit your core work today. It's a must. Add in finishers as needed.

Dynamic Effort Upper Day

You can probably guess where we are going here by now. Pick a movement, like bench press. Let's go 9×3. Week 1 is at 60 percent, Week 2 at 65 percent, Week 3 at 70 percent, and Week 4 at 75 percent. However, let's break up the 9×3 sets. The first 3×3 will be with a close grip. The next 3×3 will be with a wide grip. The last 3×3 will be with a grip between the close and wide grip. You can repeat this process for several months before changing things. Then, if you want, do the same thing with floor press for several months, and then come back. You're all set for your main lift.

Accessories are important here, like always. You'll need more sets and reps for the dynamic days too. A few things to note here: Your triceps finish any pressing movement. You cannot neglect them. Always get back work and rear deltoid (shoulder) work done. You must build up all aspects of your posterior chain.

What's Missing?

The template and philosophy above are the basic guidelines for your Training. You should search out and read more books to expand your Knowledge. There are full textbooks on the topic alone. But even the template above has holes in it. You must use some other guiding principles to help you determine when to add in more work.

No Weaknesses

No part of your body should be neglected or weak. None. Any weakness will lower your ability to perform your sport at the highest level. Period. Any significant weakness or imbalance will increase your chance for injury. At the end of the day, you are responsible for you. Hunt and fix your weaknesses. So, if your grip strength is lacking, work on it. Weak arms and neck? Add those Accessories in for the next six months. Haven't done any calf training? Calf raises must be added to the program.

Other than a barbell, one of the best tools is a sled. Pushing and pulling any resistance makes the entire body work, so moving any sleds or carrying any objects are great for building overall raw strength. I love both options immensely.

What about the other three days in the week? You can add in work here. Use those sessions to address your lagging muscle groups and weaknesses. Core work can be done again. Do not be overly taxing on those days. Your four main days are the priority. It's not how hard can you train. It's how hard can you train, recover fully, and train hard again, every day. If you cannot recover for your next main day, then you're doing more damage than good.

Reminder: You must remember the Pyramid. If you want to grow a section of it, then you must grow the support below it. For example, if you clean 190 lb. and front squat 190 lb., then you cannot clean any heavier weight until you can front squat a heavier weight. The strength (front squat) must lead and be larger than the speed or power (clean). In addition, the size of the total pyramid must grow for you to grow. Meaning, you will have to do more work and volume to squat 405 lb. than what you did to squat 225 lb. The Pyramid can only be as tall as its base.

What If You Have A Coach?

This is a great first step. Follow his or her guidance and work your butt off with what he or she asks you to do. Also recognize that no one is perfect. Everyone is flawed. I am especially flawed. And so is your coach. Also recognize that any leader, coach, parent is trying to govern the group, team, or family for their overall best interest. This normal and necessary dynamic creates imperfections in coaching the team. What does this mean? It means that what the team is doing may or may not be optimal for you at this moment. That's fine and okay. It's expected. Still follow your coach and do your best.

However, it still takes what it takes. You are still responsible for you. You must still fill in the gaps and holes in your Training. You must still hunt your weaknesses. This does *not* give you a pass to be weak in an area. You do not get a pass and get to have major imbalances leading to injury. This is still America, and you are still responsible for you. Own everything!

Problem: Your coach only focuses on speed and power. Solution: You must add in accessories that build your strength. Then you must assess and build your absolute strength on the side. This is very, very challenging. You'll need an outside coach to help you with this.

Problem: Your coach only develops the front (anterior) parts of your body. Solution: You must add in accessories that build your back side (posterior).

Problem: Your core is weak and unstable. Solution: You must add in core strengthening training to fix the issue.

Problem: You're a baseball or softball player, and your coach is trying to ruin you with all your innings pitched and play in the field. In addition, your coach is trying to ruin you with all your practices and zero strength training. Solution: Improve your grip strength. Improve your shoulder and scapula strength to help prevent injury. Improve you core strength. Improve your rotational strength. Improve your leg strength for leg-drive when pitching and swinging. You're probably low on time.

Solution: Get off your phone! Get your homework done immediately after school. Dominate at practice. Eat a ton of protein and get to bed early. Train from 6:00 a.m. to 7:00 a.m. before school starts. There is a solution to every problem. You're not busy. You're undisciplined and don't have a plan. Now prioritize and execute.

Problem: Your training at the high school involves seventy-five kids at the same time with one coach. Solution: Get it done as best you can at school. And find another gym to train at to fix and fill the gaps in your training on your own.

Problem: Your college S&C coach only focuses on speed. You don't get nearly enough volume for you to improve. He runs you too much with suboptimal conditioning. This scenario is very typical. How do you know it's a problem? Have your main benchmark numbers improved significantly over a year's time? If not. . . huge red flag and problem. Solution: Get a coach to guide you remotely to fill in the gaps. You may have to go to the college rec center to get more work done. You may need a different gym all-together in the summer. It depends. But it still takes what it takes. Appeal to your coach or coaches. Find a way. Once you're playing in college, you're one step away from playing in the pros. You're so close. This is your shot. You must be Relentless and capitalize on it. And it's not that your coach is a bad dude. He's trying to prepare the entire team as best he can. Do not get lulled into the idea that what you're doing is all you need to do. Build your body so it can dominate.

Training For Your Sport

Training for your sport is about things you must do in the weight room that will help you in your sport. "How" and "when" are great questions to ask about the timing of implementation. Here's the deal, the straight dope: Grade school and middle school require none of this. Simply become well-rounded, stronger, and faster. Speed can be built quickly and lost quickly. Strength building takes a lifetime to complete.

Build both, but focus a little more on strength earlier on at this time. How much more? Seventy-thirty strength-speed.

High school: Keep doing what you're doing. Ideally, you're playing two sports at this point. One is your main sport, and the other is complementary. Stick to this approach. Ask any college coach when they're recruiting you. Playing two sports is best. As for your training, keep the same well-rounded approach for at least the first two years and most likely three. Halfway into your junior year, start being more specific about what you're trying to build. This is the time you'll be recruited most. Going into your senior year, you must fully dominate. All-state is the minimum target if you want to play in college. You must be the best in your conference at your position, if not the state. Approach it that way.

Once you're in college, you're getting close to the big time. With NIL deals around, you are a brand and an asset. You must treat your day and training like a full-time business. No questions about it. Or you just don't have it. It starts right after your senior year season ends. Take two weeks off, then block everything out. Prepare for college Relentlessly now!

Example: My son Jack had the painful experience of graduating in 2021 in the height of COVID-19. That meant no visiting D1 schools. All planned visits were canceled. He was lucky to have a season at all. ("Senior Day" was Week 1 because it wasn't clear there would be Week 2.) He was just sending videos, emails, and DMs to coaches all the time. Each school only had about one-third of the normal annual roster spots available. This was because the NCAA granted an extra year of eligibility to current college athletes. What a waste. Jack's senior class was essentially told they weren't needed. So, he finished his fall semester in high school, and normally he'd have had track in the spring. Not this time. He left that team and focused on his training and recruiting. The goals were clear: Continue to raise all his lifts; lower all his speed test times; put out videos of him being a badass athlete; send all the videos to coaches. He played both ways and special teams his senior year (WR,

OLB, and kick and punt). He ate everything in sight and struggled to keep his weight above 205 lb. at six-foot-one. But he trained year-round with me for years. Lifting year-round is the only way to be great. But in the spring, he really had to ramp it up. I found him a couple great training partners: Clay Peters was a strong hard-nosed rugby guy who trained with us. He went on to play at Marian University. Gavin Ritter was a wide receiver who trained with us. He just finished at DePauw University. For context, these were Jack's numbers by the end of spring:

- Weighed 207 lb.
- Back squat: 500 lb.
- Bench press: 315 lb.
- Power clean: 300 lb.
- Max strict pull-ups: Fifteen
- Legless rope climbs: Check
- Seated box jump: 42″
- Standing broad jump: 9′6″
- Five-ten-five drill: 4.21 laser
- Forty-yard dash: 4.79 hand

Jack received a preferred walk-on (PWO) offer from Ball State University in January 2021. It wasn't obvious they wanted him. How do we know? Jack messaged BSU coaches seventeen times before his first response. Seven emails and ten DMs on Twitter. He was truly at the bottom of the list. It didn't matter if he was all-state, all-conference, academic all-state, etc. It was easily a supply/demand issue. There wasn't the demand for as many athletes because the supply was full. Nationwide, the recruited athletes went down. Didn't matter. He got his PWO, and now the stakes just went up. Good.

You don't have to get ready if you stay ready. Jack was told he would join the team in January 2022 after his first fall semester. All right. Great. Let's train. Bigger, faster, stronger. Fast forward to June of 2021 and he gets "the call." He was moved up and invited to summer camp and the fall 2022 season. No slack. That's why you must be Relentless. As Charles Darwin proved, survival isn't simply to the strongest or the smartest. It's to the one that adapts the best. Train your butt off and put a huge hurt on the opposition. It was a good thing he kept his training up and didn't slack. His start date was just moved up five months. Let's go.

Training For Your Sport Examples

Take Tyler Miller, a thrower for Purdue University (shot put and discus). He was ranked number two in the Big Ten. If you look at the throwing motion, throwers get a lot of return if they are outstanding in the "hang" position. That means they are great with hang cleans and hang snatches. I asked him about his deadlift, and his answer made a lot of sense. He told me he couldn't deadlift 500 lb. off the floor. But from above the knee, he could pull 835 lb. Lesson: yes, it's great to perform a full range of motion lift. But at the elite level, who cares?! What translates to your sport most? He was already well-rounded and strong. Now he's trying to win a title and qualify for the Olympics. It was optimal for him to be strong pulling a bar from above the knee. So that's what he did.

Let's say that you play football on the offensive line. When your hands shoot forward, the motion more closely mimics a close grip bench press than a wide grip bench press. Ideally, it's most like a Swiss bar bench press. Answer: Do more close-grip bench press. Get stronger in that position. It will translate better to your sport.

Athletes in most sports move forward, backward, and laterally side-to-side. Problem: They don't get stronger laterally often enough, only forward and backward. Laterally, they are weaker. Answer: Add in sumo deadlift and wide-stance box squats to address the deficiency. Work on this for six to nine months and see how much more powerful you are when you must push and change direction violently.

Maybe you play soccer, where there can be a decent amount of contact. Or you play lacrosse, where there also is a decent amount of contact. Does it really help you to have big arms? Well, it depends. Does it help you play better? It helps some. Does it help protect your radius, ulna, and humerus (arm bones) from impact injuries? Yes. Answer: Still get bigger arms to help protect yourself.

Or maybe you play a contact sport, and concussions are a real threat. Answer: Build up your neck, upper shoulders, and trap muscles. Those muscles will help brace your neck from the whiplash effects from contact.

Or say you're a setter in volleyball. Problem: You arch your lower back while getting into position to set the ball. Your lower lumbar region is severely compromised. Answer: Make the area and area around it ironclad strong. That means a lot of reverse hypers for your back to heal. Strengthen your glutes and hamstrings with heavy bridges and leg curls. Strengthen your lower back with back extensions and good mornings. Create a solid core with dead bugs, heavy plank holds, and oblique holds.

We can go on and on here. At the highest level, you will need to focus more of your efforts specializing your training. It's not nearly necessary early on. But near college and beyond, it becomes critical. Find a coach. Train accordingly.

Quick Note

There is overlap with the six Inch Blocks. Your Knowledge with respect to your Training must grow as you evolve as an athlete. Everything matters. Andre Agassi was recounting his tennis days against Boris Becker. Agassi noticed a facial "tell" from Becker. Becker's tongue would poke out his mouth in the direction he was about to serve the ball. Agassi noticed it and capitalized on it for years. This elite level of Knowledge must be sought after in your Training.

Example: It's not just knowing how to squat correctly. It's finding the weaknesses in your squat technique. It's finding the weaknesses in your squat strength. Then it's finding the accessories to fix your squat. Then it's teaching your Teammates the same lessons. Then it's fixing the issues with your Teammates and training them to fix yours.

Then it's applied to the skills on the field and Training there. Dennis Rodman would simply watch how the basketball would bounce off the rim and backboard based on the angle of the shots. It was a clue for him to rebound better. That time, effort and dedication were sport-specific Training. It helped him become the best rebounder of his time.

Once again, the more relentless you apply your efforts and maximize your time, the better you'll perform. Kaizen. Get one Inch better every day.

CHAPTER 31

TRAINING - WAY OF INCHES

Process is king. Let's look at, analyze, and improve your Training process. This is the grind. This is your work. This is what you do after you fuel and prepare yourself for the daily tests and battles. This is the brutal regimen you put yourself through to improve. When you know your "Why," then this is what you do because of your "Why." You must train hard. And then you must Recover hard. Then you can train hard again. Be Relentless. Look at your Training Block and be honest with yourself. Then, let's find ways to get better immediately.

TRAINING

Strength

- 10 Points: You are in the top 10 percent (in strength) at your position nationwide.
- 8 Points: You are in the top 10 percent in your conference.
- 6 Points: You are in the top 10 percent of your position group on team.
- 4 Points: You are in the top 20 percent of your position group on the team.
- 2 Points: You are in the top 50 percent of your position group on the team.

- 0 Points: All else.

POINTS: _____

Fastest and Most Powerful

- 10 Points: You are in the top 10 percent (in speed and power) at your position nationwide.
- 8 Points: You are in the top 10 percent in your conference.
- 6 Points: You are in the top 10 percent of your position group on the team.
- 4 Points: You are in the top 20 percent of your position group on the team.
- 2 Points: You are in the top 50 percent of your position group on the team.
- 0 Points: All else.

POINTS: _____

Stamina

- 10 Points: You are in the top 10 percent (in stamina) at your position nationwide.
- 8 Points: You are in the top 10 percent in your conference.
- 6 Points: You are in the top 10 percent of your position group on the team.
- 4 Points: You are in the top 20 percent of your position group on the team.
- 2 Points: You are in the top 50 percent of your position group on the team.
- 0 Points: All else.

POINTS: _____

Resiliency (You're the Toughest.)

- 10 Points: You are in the top 10 percent (in resiliency) at your position nationwide.
- 8 Points: You are in the top 10 percent in your conference.
- 6 Points: You are in the top 10 percent of your position group on the team.
- 4 Points: You are in the top 20 percent of your position group on the team.
- 2 Points: You are in the top 50 percent of your position group on the team.
- 0 Points: All else.

POINTS: _____

Offseason

- 10 Points: You put in the most work of anyone on your team (in the gym and on the field, doing everything physical to improve).
- 8 Points: You are in the top ten people on your team for putting in the most work.
- 6 Points: You put in the most work of anyone in your position group.
- 0 Points: All else.

POINTS: _____

In-season

- 10 Points: You put in the most work of anyone on your team (in the gym and on the field, doing everything physical to improve).

- 8 Points: You are in the top ten people on your team for putting in the most work.
- 6 Points: You put in the most work of anyone in your position group.
- 0 Points: All else.

POINTS: _____

Kaizen

- 10 Points: You have a process for improving and adhere to it without fail.
- 8 Points: You mostly have a process and adhere to it.
- 5 Points: You occasionally have a process and adhere to it.
- 0 Points: All else.

POINTS: _____

Training Mentor

- 10 Points: You have one and connect weekly.
- 8 Points: You have one and connect monthly.
- 5 Points: You have one and connect quarterly.
- 0 Points: All else.

POINTS: _____

How effectively are you working with a Training accountability ally (or allies)?

- 10 Points: You and your ally review your results weekly, enforce a "carrot/stick," and adjust.

- 7 Points: You and your ally review your results monthly and sometimes enforce "carrot/stick."
- 4 Points: You and your ally review your results quarterly.
- 0 Points: All else.

POINTS: _____

You know your number one Training Strength (Competitive Advantage):

- 10 points. Otherwise: 0 points.

POINTS: _____

You know your number one Training Weakness (Weak Link):

- 10 points. Otherwise: 0 points.

POINTS: _____

You know your number one Training Opportunity (Target):

- 10 points. Otherwise: 0 points.

POINTS: _____

You know your number one Training Threat (Enemy):

- 10 points. Otherwise: 0 points.

POINTS: _____

TOTAL POINTS: _____

OVERALL AVERAGE (TOTAL POINTS /13) _____

This assessment presents some new challenges. The obvious question is this: How do I know how I compare with other athletes nationwide, or in my conference? On the surface, it's hard to say. It's not an exact science. However, in some cases, numbers are published everywhere all the time. Or are they? This is where leaning on the Knowledge of your coach will be critical for your success. And it would take some digging and detective work so you and your coach can uncover the answers. Ultimately there will need to be some estimates made. It could even take some guess work too.

What can you discover on your own? Let's work through an example. Football has an easy way of finding information. Go to www.nfl.com and you can find the results of the 2023 NFL combine and sort by the position. Looking at linebackers, we can learn and calculate the following:

TEST	BEST SCORE	WORST SCORE	AVERAGE	TOP 1/3 SCORE
FORTY-YARD DASH	4.39 sec.	4.69 sec.	4.545 sec.	4.46 sec.
TEN-YARD SPLIT	1.52 sec.	1.69 sec.	1.569 sec.	1.528 sec.
VERTICAL JUMP	38.5"	30.5"	33.83"	36.6"
BROAD JUMP	10'9"	9'4"	10.19'	10.65'
THREE-CONE DRILL	6.74 sec.	7.32 sec.	7.084 sec.	6.852 sec.
SHUTTLE DRILL	4.24 sec.	4.43 sec.	4.365 sec.	4.297 sec.
BENCH PRESS	29 reps	15 reps	22.3 reps	27.09 reps

I simply used Google to find the information. Then I put all the data in a spreadsheet to find the averages and one standard deviation. (One standard deviation, roughly, tells me that the top third, or 33 percent, of scores were that number or better.) All right, well now we have some-thing to work toward.

Next questions: What other scores are useful to know? Height? Weight? Power clean? Back squat? Weighted plank hold? Grip strength? Maybe yes, maybe no. Ask your team's strength and conditioning coach. Get some guidance. Then you can start to piece together what the optimal player looks like and can do physically. Those become tar-gets.

Improving your Training process is the goal. The targets are just things you measure along the way. (Example: Your target is to have a two times body weight squat. Measure the sets, reps, and weight you do to help you obtain that target.) You really must measure your process work. (Example: You trained your lower body three times a week for seventy-five minutes each time. And track your sets, reps, and weight.) Your "normal" practice and training is the mandatory work. Your "hard" work begins with what you do in addition to the required train-ing. Everyone else is doing the required work. That's the minimum. That is *not* you! You do the maximum! This is your Training Block goal.

Example: A big weakness is your back strength. Your Training Block goal is to accomplish sixty to eighty extra chin-ups or pull-ups twice a week. And twice a week, you'll also accomplish 120–160 extra rows (barbell rows, single arm rows, seated rows, ring rows). You'll do this for six weeks and retest your back strength. Then you'll decide to continue, add reps, change reps, or focus on another group. It takes what it takes. The hard part is that if you want more of something, then you must do more. You must grow your Training Pyramid.

Regardless of your sport, you must work to find the same metrics and targets. If you know nothing else about the metrics and targets for your sport, then your goal is to be the strongest, fastest, most powerful kid on your team. That's the minimum. Be the best on your team. It's a solid target if you know nothing else.

Back to your Assessment Test. You see your score. Retest yourself at the end of every quarter of the year (March 31, June 30, September

30, December 31). Ask yourself a series of reflective questions and gauge your progress over the last quarter.

- What is your level of Knowledge on optimizing your Training? Do you know the basics and have a general understanding of what it takes to perform and improve?
- What have your habits been? Can you quantify what's required to compete at a high level?
- Who has been a solid Training Teammate and who has not? Whom should you add or eliminate?
- What are your next steps to level up your Kaizen approach to your process?

SWOT analysis. This time apply your SWOT analysis to the Training Block. Be sure to prioritize and identify your Competitive Advantage and your Weak Link. You must advance in these areas to optimize your performance. Write out your process goals and habits for the next quarter. What is your number one Target for this quarter? Share with your Training accountability ally. Devise your carrot and stick for your check-ins. Bring on a mentor as well. I can't imagine a scenario where you work this diligently and don't advance. It's impossible. You'll continue to crush it.

- Strength:
    - List them all.
    - What are your top three?
    - What is your number one Strength (Competitive Advantage)?
- Weaknesses:
    - List them all.
    - What are your top three?
    - What is your number one Weakness (Weak Link)?
- Opportunities:

- ◦ List them all.
- ◦ What are your top three?
- ◦ What is your number one Opportunity (Target)?
- Threats:
  - ◦ List them all.
  - ◦ What are your top three?
  - ◦ What is your number one Threat (Enemy)?

Training Way of Inches

This is where the rubber meets the road. What matters most is what you do. What work do you put in? What can you accomplish physically on the field or court? Athletes are assets that perform a function. What can you do physically that impacts the team and gives the team the edge to win? This is what we are after here.

Get your Mindset right here. It must be that you put in massive amounts of extra work to get ahead and win. Get your tribe of Teammates right here too. That means your Training partners. That also means you coaches. You must plead your case incessantly and respectfully, so they push your body, so it maximizes your output. Get your coaches to create the best physical version of you possible. And then do some more.

Get constant, consistent, and precise feedback on what you need to improve. Hunt weaknesses. Build your Pyramid until you physically dominate the field or court. Identify your obstacles and work around them. Some pros have home gyms so they can get more work done. Some college kids get extra Training equipment or go to the rec center to get more work done. Write down the obstacles and come up with solutions. Then reassess a million times until you retire for good.

10 Training Habits

Not sure where to begin or overwhelmed? Don't be. I got you. Look at the ten basic habits listed below. Pick one and move forward. Consistency is what matters. Keep at it daily.

1. Are you completely uncertain of what to do? Just spend an extra thirty minutes daily in the gym. Ask your coach for something you can work on and measure that. Ask for different things to do daily. Do that for six weeks and reassess.
2. Strengthen your posterior (back side) every time you train. Most programs lack this component. So, it's easy to make an impact here.
3. Everyone benefits from a stronger core. Work up to a weighted plank hold of 1× your bodyweight for one minute.
4. Spend twenty minutes with a mobility app prior to each training session. Getting your body into the right position is critical for moving the maximum weight.
5. Video record your lifts. Then you can see what's wrong and what's breaking down. Ask your coach for input.
6. Develop a huge-ass box squat. Squatting is the best day of the week and cures a lot of sins. This is gold.
7. Push the intensity with your accessories. No failed reps, but push hard here. This is where you make your money.
8. Learn a ton! Read and watch everything on Training. Ask questions all the time.
9. Take notes on your Training. Quantify everything. Push to set records in all aspects.
10. Have fun making it competitive with your Teammates. Get them better and push them. It'll get you better in the process.

<u>Scan the following QR code</u> or visit: https://athlete-builder.com to access and download the assessment in this chapter and other resources (free nutrition resources and free workout programs).

CHAPTER 32

NUTRITION

H ave you ever heard any of the following statements?

You are what you eat.
You can't outwork a bad diet.
Two-thirds of your success is Nutrition.
You must eat to perform.

Yes. Me too. The thing is they are all true. No kidding. Absolutely true. There are countless books and programs for eating. There is no lack of methodologies. Here are some rules you must follow for continued success.

- Rule 1: The best plan is the one you stick to.
- Rule 2: Sustainability. Select sustainable habits. Do *not* select quick-fix or gimmick habits. This is true with everything and definitely true with your Nutrition.
- Rule 3: Process is king.

What's my journey been like? A severe roller coaster. I played racquetball for three years in high school and for two years in college at Purdue University. I was 6′3″ and 190 lb. at age fourteen and stayed the same for the next five years. Unfortunately, I destroyed my back while playing at Purdue, which ended my career by age twenty-one. I graduated at 260 lb., mostly fat. I stayed at that weight for about fifteen years before deciding to get my act together. I had enough one day at a weight of 280 lb. So, I went the P90X training route (home workouts on DVD with my own body weight and bands) and added running. Then I advanced to group training six months later which then evolved to CrossFit. My weight dropped below 220 lb. while I ran a sub-two-hour half marathon (13.1 miles). I was lean but not strong. Once I opened Unbreakable (March 2013), I started learning more about powerlifting and eventually strongman competing. The next six years (2014–2020) I packed on plenty of muscle but also plenty of fat. I topped out at 319 lb. and 34 percent fat. I had a 600+ lb. deadlift, 300+ lb./hand farmers carry, pressed 300 lb. overhead, and carried 800 lb. on my back with a yoke. And then in 2020, at the age of forty-five, my body told me that my time competing in amateur strongman was over. That year I broke my foot, tore ligaments in my wrist, ruptured a couple discs in my back, and had a blood clot. Yes. It was time to change again.

As of this writing I'm down to 260 lb. with 23 percent body fat. Currently, I don't move weight over 300 lb. because of being on blood thinners. Excessive straining could lead to leaking blood through different vessels. And it turns out that wouldn't be good if it occurred in my brain. The good news is that along the way, I experienced being a multitude of different kinds of athletes. Each version of myself had different Nutrition and Training requirements. Some versions were good; others were better; and some were terrible.

And over ten years at Unbreakable Athletics, we have seen and coached a couple thousand athletes too. Once we take in all the data from those athletes and my own life experiences, add in the nutrition courses, and talk with other experts and coaches, we have the processes for you to perform with your eating.

We will look at many different factors and techniques in your Nutrition. There are the basics to go over, like calories, macronutrients, hydration, and supplements. We will explore what it takes for "hard gainers" and those with "gifted bodies." We will also look at game-day preparations and execution. We will touch on recovery but address it further in the Recovery section of the book. Finally, we will outline the priorities and the process for developing your own personal plan for performance.

Here is a quick example. Brian Shaw, four-time World's Strongest Man. He's 6'7" and 440 lb. Michael Phelps is the most decorated Olympian ever with twenty-eight medals. He is 6'4" and 198 lb. Both are completely different athletes in completely different sports. What's staggering is that both also consumed 12,000–14,000 calories per day when training. For context, a McDonald's Big Mac has 550 calories. One slice of Pizza Hut hand-tossed meat lover's pizza has about 300 calories. To get to 12,000 calories would take twenty-two Big Macs or forty slices of pizza. Clearly, it's more on the 14,000 calorie days. That's each day as well. If you're like me, you're now wondering how many trips to the bathroom happen each day too! The answer is too many. But there is a way to do it. And ultimately it takes what it takes to do the things you want to do. For them and athletes like them it becomes calories/bite. Chewing alone is a huge challenge. There is no getting around it. But they both found a way to get it done in completely different sports. You must too. This is how.

CHAPTER 33

NUTRITION - BASICS WITHOUT FOOD

Let's be clear about a few things. The answer to most every question or issue you have when it comes to performing as an athlete (or for that matter anything else) is "It depends." It really does. This will not be a high-level book on Nutrition. Why? Because that would be an entire book unto itself. What we outline and teach you here will cover 90–95+ percent of what you need. For most, if not all of you, it will be meaningful enough to get you to your 95–97 percent. And let's be real, a lot of you are such terrible eaters (the whole world is—and me included at one time), that what we do here alone will change your life forever.

At the end of the Nutrition section, we will outline a process for success for you. Remember, apply the fundamentals like a champion, and you have your best shot. Concentrate on the habits that move the needle the most.

There are two approaches that are seemingly diametrically opposed. On the one hand, you have the James Clear *Atomic Habits* school of thought: Start small. Increase systematically and consistently. Make new habits obvious, attractive, easy, and satisfying.

Then you have the Jim Beebe/Grant Cardone/Tim Grover school of thought: all in or not at all.

So, which is it? The answer is both. Start small and be strategic and systematic. And keep improving and evolving Relentlessly until you are at the top, looking down from the mountain of greatness. Reach for your best potential and let the world know you conquered yourself and are reaching your fullest potential.

Commit. Commit to improving this Block for you as an athlete. Let your accountability ally know where you're going and "tribe up." Keep your closest allies in the loop about what you're doing and where you're going. Keep each other in line and beyond. Push each other. Remind yourself of your "Why." And you probably have more than one by now. Keep this top of mind. Post them everywhere: the fridge, your bathroom mirror, on your car dashboard, with your phone alarms, your computer screensaver, tattooed on your body. As you set goals stick to the process: SMART (Specific, Measurable, Attainable, Relevant, Time Sensitive).

You can't improve a habit until you have the habit. How do you start? You start with what do you eat and drink? Every athlete we coach starts with this question. What goes in your mouth? This is where Integrity comes in. Some athletes will be embarrassed to disclose what they eat. Well, no one has time for that obstacle. We are only effective when working with the truth. You have two options. The suboptimal option but still effective is to write down in a notebook (paper or electronically) everything you consume. And I mean everything. A handful of seven M&Ms counts. Four sixteen-ounce glasses of water or beer also counts. If you take fish oil as a supplement, there are calories there too. Inches: Everything matters. Some things matter more than others. However, first you need to know what you're consuming. A better way is to use an app like My Fitness Pal (MFP). It's free and the upgrade service is worthwhile and reasonable. It's great that MFP lists and quantifies the calories, macros, and micros for you. It saves you a lot of math when calculating your numbers. It's not perfect, but it is quite helpful.

You must do this for a week to get a baseline. The more you track, the better you do. Most find this habit tedious and not sustainable. Consequently, we don't push this on our athletes until they are ready and at that level. However, occasionally we must track numbers for a week to get more accurate in our approach. Don't worry. You won't need to do this every week. You can build up to this level and make enormous progress along the way.

There are a few other basic pieces of data you'll need to start improving. What are your eating habits and times currently? Does Mom make everything? Do you have team meals? Do you have dorm food or cook on your own? Do you skip meals? (Never be this idiot.) Do you have any idea at all how to cook and prepare? Which meals are your largest? Smallest? How fast do you eat? Do you eat like a five-year-old (pasta and chicken fingers only)? Do you bring the right snacks everywhere you go? Do you have back-up supplies in your car or room? Take a moment and give yourself an honest assessment of where you are with your Nutrition Block. Ask an objective ally to be critical of you. This way is so much easier to make improvements. Be brutally honest with where you are starting.

Then, where do you want to go? Clearly this is just as important as where you are. If you have no path or target, then any direction will do. Do not be a rudderless ship. Where do you want to go? Words are important. Where *must* you go? Lose ten pounds of fat? Twenty pounds? Lose ten pounds of fat and gain ten pounds of muscle? Take your body fat from 24.5 percent to 14 percent? Add enough muscle to squat 600 lb. and run a sub-4.5 forty-yard dash? Get strong enough to bench 225 lb. forty times at the NFL combine? Lower your body fat to 8 percent for wrestling season? Where must you go?

What gets in your way? What are your obstacles? It could be that you are unaware of how to eat. This is the main one. Or you're aware of how to eat, but you don't have a systematic process for optimizing it. This is just as critical. Perhaps you don't have the resources because you don't always control the menu if you live at home or can only eat dorm food or team meals. A consistent challenge is that you don't have the Discipline to be great. . . yet. Luckily there is a solution to every problem. Expand your mind, and you'll find solutions for your issues. If you cannot do that, then I surely can. You may not love it, but the solutions work. Then it becomes a question of how Relentlessly you apply the processes.

That's up to you. I can get you there. Will you do the work required to be Unbreakable? We'll see.

CHAPTER 34

NUTRITION - BASICS ROUND TWO

You must be aware. You must learn. You must plan.

> *Art is long, and Time is fleeting,*
> *And our hearts, though stout and brave,*
> *Still, like muffled drums, are beating*
> *Funeral marches to the grave.*
> *In the world's broad field of battle,*
> *In the bivouac of Life,*
> *Be not like dumb, driven cattle!*
> *Be a hero in the strife!*
> *– A Psalm of Life* by Henry Wadsworth Longfellow, stanzas 4 and 5

Nutritionally, your world and mine are not set up naturally to be healthy. At all! You must "Be not like dumb, driven cattle! / Be a hero in the strife!" You must be aware. You must learn. You must plan. You must rise and attack against your surroundings, habits, and Knowledge. The world is set up, made easier, and made cheaper for you to eat crap. All the time! Some areas of the country are even worse and don't have grocery stores. They have convenience stores with only processed food. Nothing in convenience stores is ever fresh. It's a real challenge because quick processed food is much cheaper. . . in the short run. In the long run, it will cost you your gains and success in your sport. In the very long run, it will cost you significantly more in health care costs, due to dependency on medication, diseases, lower quality of life, and earlier death. You must choose. Choose wisely and remain Disciplined. Hold yourself to your standard.

Awareness

What are you shoving into your mouth? You must know. Again, use an app like My Fitness Pal, a notebook or planner, or a tablet with a resource like OneNote. But whatever way you choose, you must know what you're eating. It can be an annoying step. But it's necessary, so get it done early. Then once you know what's going in, you can apply your Kaizen principle and make small tweaks and improvements to adjust. The top-level people track everything every day. You need not do that. Just do it for a week. Then make some adjustments. Then do it again a month later to see how it's working. But first you must know what's going in. Period.

Read labels. Read the math part. Pay no attention to the marketing lies. Read the math only. What are some of the lies? Subway's *Eat Fresh* is an example. The veggies are the freshest items. The breads are processed. The meats are all processed. The cheeses are processed. Then you add on fatty sauces or oils. Then the fat content is as high as a cheeseburger, and 75 percent of the food is processed, not fresh. Now, on a relative basis, it is fresher than McDonalds food. So that's a win. Is it as fresh as what you can make at home? No. The question becomes which athlete are you aspiring to become? Pretender? College? Pro? Statue? If you don't eat much at all, then shoot. Just put something in. . . Pretender. If you're always eating greasy fast food, upgrade to Subway or make your own food. If you're at the "Subway" level, then upgrade and eat what you make at home? If you're in school, you'll eat a lot of what is prepared for you. Therefore, you must supplement more and other food once you're at home to compensate for what's lacking. Either way, read the label! Figure out what's going in.

When you read the labels, do some quick math yourself. The information on the back can be wrong sometimes or misleading. Recall that protein and carbs have 4 calories/gram. Fat has 9 calories/gram. Well, the calories listed on the back of items can be miscalculated. It could be intentional or not. The intent doesn't matter. What matters is that you know what you're consuming.

Next is the serving size. Example: You buy a 22 oz. bottle of orange Gatorade and read that it has 100 calories and 27 grams of carbs, 0 grams of fat and proteins. (4 calories/gram × 27 grams = 108. Looks like Gatorade "rounded down.") You'll also need to understand if there are one or two servings in the bottle. If it's two servings, then the numbers listed are doubled if you consume the entire thing. In this case, it's one serving per bottle. The point is that reading is important. Know what's going into your body.

Eating Out

Big one here. For 95+ percent of restaurants, they want you to return solely because of the way their food tastes and your experience. There are some that want you to return because their food is healthy, tastes good, and you still have a good experience. But the overwhelming majority put all the "yummy goodness" items in the food so it tastes great. Then you'll love it and keep coming back. There is nothing wrong with that either. You still must "Be not like dumb driven cattle!" You must know what's going into your system.

Now it's more common that restaurants list the calories next to items on their menus. This habit is a huge help. It does fall short in terms of listing the macronutrients (proteins, carbs, and fats). Regardless, it's still an improvement. Now what are you to do? Prepare! Go online before you go to the restaurant. Select what you'll want to eat. Then upload the items into My Fitness Pal and see where you're at. It will be eye-opening. I remember when I was a true idiot at eating. I went to Claddaugh Irish Pub during Lent on Friday because Catholics can't eat meat except for fish, and I'm Catholic. Well, I ordered the fish and chips, thinking I'm abiding by only eating fish. Wow. That was enlightening. One serving had 77 grams of carbs, 47 grams of fat, and 29 grams of protein for 850 calories. Of course, that was for one serving. It came with two, and I ate both. That doubled all the numbers. This didn't include the sauces or any drinks I had along with it. This was one meal. I almost doubled my fat intake for the entire day. I had a good protein number. But I also almost maxed out my carbs for the day in one sitting. Moral of the story: Figure it out. Prepare in advance. Come up with a plan. Picking restaurants with purpose is a good start. Chipotle is decent for getting solid macros: meats, veggies, and rice. Then add or subtract the other items based on your goals. Then execute. You must eat to live, not live to eat.

Myths

- It's just calories in versus calories out. Yes and no. This is the basic formula for weight loss and weight gain. However, the calories in a Snickers bar are not the same as the calories in whole foods. Ask which athlete you are, then eat accordingly.
- Eat small, infrequent meals. It depends. Larger meals take longer to digest and slow you down. Smaller meals are easier and keep your metabolism working. But whether you hit your calorie and macro numbers with larger or smaller meals, you'll fuel your body the same. You'll grow and recover the same. You must choose which method works with your lifestyle and execute.
- All fats are bad. Well, clearly not, especially if you value your skin, hair, and brain for starters.
- All carbs are bad. Nope. Try to compete in your sport on fifty carbs per day. You'll see your performance tank quickly. Carbs provide energy, and you must eat to perform.
- Supplements are a waste. Not true. They are not the most important tool in the belt, but supplements are still necessary. Creatine,

vitamin D, fish oil, and probiotics are great ways to help you improve your performance.

- Consume protein right after training. Not exactly. Simple carbs like a banana are best within twenty to thirty minutes of training. Forty minutes to one hour after training is the time to add in protein. The carbs will absorb and digest quickly, helping the body recover. Then the slower-digesting protein comes in to help the muscles rebuild and repair.

Water

Other than air, water is the most critical. You can go seventy-two hours without water, but not much more without really falling apart. You can go longer without food. Water allows cells to grow, flushes out waste, lubricates joints, helps convert food, regulates body temperature, and delivers oxygen. It's critical.

What's the math? For a basic rule of thumb, women should have 90 oz. and men 125 oz. per day. Another equation is your (BMR + activity level) × 1.25 mL. Both are very general equations and good starting points. Here's the easiest process. (Process is king.) Look at your urine throughout the day. Don't count your first urine sample in the morning. Then check out all others. If it's the color of a "light lemonade," then you're good to go. This is one of the easiest processes to keep it simple.

A more advanced method is to track and count the amount of water ounces you consume. Then evaluate and see how you feel throughout the day, after training, and after competing. Obviously the most important step is to adjust the intake accordingly. Back to the process: Simply have an empty, reusable gallon jug, and carry it with you everywhere. Drink as much of it as required for you to maintain the "light lemonade" color.

More basics: If you're thirsty, then take a drink. If there is a big day for you tomorrow physically, then have more water today. By the time the competition rolls around, it's too late. Prepare in advance. Also, really start limiting your water consumption in the later afternoon and early evening. You don't want to impact your sleep negatively by being up five times in the night to pee.

Electrolytes. They regulate your nerves and muscles, hydration, blood pressure, and rebuild damaged tissues. The most common examples are sodium, potassium, and calcium. That's one of the reasons I started to eat a banana after training. You need the electrolytes to hold the water in your system, especially during hot and humid conditions. If you're sweating profusely and you're consuming only water, you'll urinate a lot and continue to sweat. The combination will further dehydrate you. Drink some Gatorade, consume salt, salty snacks, or veggies. It'll help hold the water in.

Example: I was competing at the University of Kentucky in an amateur Strongman contest in 2019. It was a long day and went for twelve hours. In strongman, each event is close to your max weight for the event for between thirty and seventy-five seconds of max reps. Waiting around all day in the heat was worse than the actual events. It was late in the day and Atlas stones was my last event. I had been sweating a lot and started getting cold. Jessica Fithen was the reigning World's Strongest Woman who trained at my gym. She was there helping coach me. I asked her what was going on. I was getting chills and feeling cold while it was very hot inside the arena. And I was sweating profusely. She quickly informed me that I was getting dehydrated. In a pinch, all I could find were some salt packets at the concession stand. I quickly consumed those and about ten or fifteen minutes later, I was immediately better. It was like I was a different person. This is obviously not a great way to consume electrolytes. But you do what you must do in a bind. Live and learn. Be better-prepared next time. (Side note: I won the stones event and took second overall in the master's division. The trophy was a medieval sword. Cool!)

Supplements

Supplements are another tool in the belt. They can get you your last 5–10 percent of return from supplements, tops. These aren't the biggest tools in the belt but important nonetheless. One issue is that supplements are not regulated by the Food and Drug Administration. (Take the FDA for what it's worth.) However, it is valuable to look on the label for a third-party verification. Informed Choice is a good example of a third-party validator. Since supplements are not regulated, the industry is notorious for lying on the ingredients of their products. Therefore, buy from reputable sources and stick to the basics. And like anything else, read the label and scrutinize it so you know exactly what you're consuming. To make matters more serious, the NCAA, pro leagues, WADA, the Olympics, etc. have lists of banned substances. You must prepare and know what you're consuming. That's nothing new, just worth repeating.

The following are the five main supplements we recommend. Of course, there are others that are worthwhile. As an athlete, you're trying to maximize your performance now! These five will cover most of what you're looking for without an inordinate amount of cost.

- Vitamin D: It improves your mood and aids the immune system. It also aids in bone health, fat loss, and muscle growth.
- Fish oil: It helps get you the optimal ratio of omega-3s and omega-6s. Fish oil has anti-inflammatory properties while lowering the risk of heart disease. There is also the added boost to brain function and improved joint health.
- Probiotic: Gut health is important for simply impacting how you feel. Combining a probiotic and a prebiotic will optimize your body's ability to absorb macro- and micronutrients. Look for probiotics that contain various strains of lactobacillus bacteria.

- Whey protein: Focus on the isolates that do not contain lactose if possible. Protein is crucial for several functions especially for growing and repairing muscles. It is also challenging to consume enough protein for athletes to hit their daily numbers. Consuming a protein shake will help considerably. Of course, real food is better than a shake, but life isn't perfect. And we must make choices. Be careful here. Scrutinize the label and the company's reputation. There have been plenty of examples of fraud in this area of the industry.
- Creatine: This is one of the most widely researched supplements. The results and consensus are overwhelmingly clear: Get it and consume it. Take it daily regardless of when you train. The timing of taking it is not nearly that important. You simply want it in your system every day. The recommended dosage is 5–6 grams per day. We take 8–10 grams per day. Anything more than that will not be utilized by the body. Creatine is fantastic for greater muscle growth and strength from resistance training. It increases muscle creatine stores, water stores, and glycogen stores which all aid muscle growth.

CHAPTER 35

NUTRITION - MACRONUTRIENTS

A gain, *temet nosce*. Know thyself. If you eat like an idiot, here's the simple directive: Stop eating like an idiot. You will win more battles and see more gains. What does "eat like an idiot" mean? Here are some basic, terrible practices I see high school and college kids do all the time, including my own kids. The following are examples. Stop doing these:

- Skipping meals.
- No protein at a meal.
- The meal is only processed food.
- Not drinking water throughout the day.
- Never eating fruit or vegetables.
- Alcohol is your meal.

Change these habits first, and you can make a huge dent in what you're trying to accomplish. Let's advance further in how to eat. The following are the next level of basic for you to apply.

Calories

Yes. calories in versus calories out is a way to manage weight gain and weigh loss. This is a very low-level approach. However, it still holds true in a lot of ways. You will need to reduce your intake by (about) 3,500 calories for you to lose one pound of weight. The same holds true if you want to gain a pound of weight. You'll need to be cognizant of this fact depending on your goals. The limitation is that not all calories are equal. Consuming 3,500 calories of lean meats, fruits, and vegetables, etc. does *not* equal 3,500 calories of processed food, alcohol, candy, etc. The equation holds true but does not account for everything necessary for optimal improvement.

The next question in the iteration is what kind of weight do you need to change for your sport? For some it is lose fat. For some it is to gain muscle. For some it is to lose fat and gain muscle. For some it is to gain muscle and gain fat. The answer is it depends. Depending on your needs you'll need to know the basics of macronutrients to give yourself the best shot of eating better.

Protein

The main jobs for protein are to build and repair muscle. Protein also aids in building and maintaining bones and skin. It is critical to consume enough protein to build the body required to perform at the highest level in your sport. Protein comes in many forms: meat, dairy, some plants, nuts and legumes, and synthetically in powders and shakes. The "math" involved with protein is that 1 gram (g) of protein = 4 calories. That means that if you need 200 g of protein daily, then that will put you at 800 calories assuming the food you're consuming has zero carbohydrates and zero fat. That of course is impossible. Then you'll have to account for those calories as well.

For the most part, animal protein is a much better source than plant protein. This is especially true if you need large amounts of protein in your diet. Plant protein simply doesn't provide very much. Beef is great but could be high in fat. Fish and chicken are excellent too. Dairy is a good source as well.

For most people, a good target is to consume one gram of protein for every pound of lean muscle mass. Then you adjust up or down based on your goals. If you're trying to get stronger or bigger, then increase your intake to 1.2–1.3 g protein/pound of lean muscle mass. If you want to lose weight, then consume below the 1:1 ratio. This way you have a good starting point. Then track and see. Based on what you consume and how your train and recover, how is your body changing? Figure that out and adjust up or down accordingly.

Protein shakes: For the most part whey protein and whey protein isolate (my favorite) are optimal to consume during the day or after training. Of course, note the type of milk you use because milk contains protein as well. Whey and isolate are easy to consume and quickly absorbed, making them ideal for your body. Casein protein is best to take right before bedtime. Casein is much slower to absorb and takes longer to break down. Therefore, casein is ideal right before you sleep for seven to nine hours and your body is essentially fasting. (Breakfast = Break + Fast.)

Amounts? Do not overload meals with too much protein. Do not do this even if you must hit large numbers of daily protein either (300–400+ g protein/day). Why not? The body simply will not utilize it all. Once you get forty to sixty grams of protein in a meal, that's about it for that digestive cycle. You'll need multiple meals and/or snacks throughout the day for you to get your numbers in. If you take in much larger amounts in one sitting, your body will either convert more of it to fat or more likely, it'll send it through as waste.

With all macronutrients, nothing is utilized fully or perfectly. Similarly, there is no perfect food. Most protein is utilized for your muscles. A much smaller amount will be converted and used for energy. By the same token, some will not be used and stored as fat. Lastly, some won't be converted and will be eliminated as waste. The food isn't perfect. The body isn't perfect. And the way your body absorbs and utilizes protein will not be the same way someone else absorbs and utilizes protein. The answers here are for most people.

As an example, I've seen guys training in my gym who are shredded, and they eat an enormous amount of protein along with an enormous amount of Oreo cookies and candy. Still others have a very clean diet but carry an extra 6–12 percent of body fat more than the Oreo guys. To make matters worse/more "fun," your level of training impacts your nutrition needs. As you age, your nutrition needs change as well as how your body handles it. I've seen a multitude of athletes consume protein shakes daily for ten years. Then once they hit age forty, they are suddenly lactose intolerant. That's annoying. So, they are forced to adjust again.

What's the answer? It depends. Like always. Take notes and see what works for you now, and keep a log. Then you'll have data. Once you have the data, then you can adjust based on what you must accomplish.

Some good protein snack examples: Greek yogurt, cottage cheese, tuna packets, string cheese, humus, some nuts (but not those high in fat).

Carbohydrates

Here is where you get most of your energy. Carbs break down into glucose to feed your cells. This provides the energy for your body and the brain. Carbs also aid in the body's ability to absorb fat. There are two distinct categories of carbohydrates: simple and complex. Simple carbs (monosaccharides) are absorbed quicker and immediately used for energy. This occurs primarily in the small intestine. There is a spike in blood sugar and a boost in energy. Carbs that are not utilized are eliminated as waste or stored as fat. The math is the same here as with protein: 1 gram of carbs = 4 calories. Examples of simple carbs are carbs found in drinks (Gatorade, pop, juices, etc.), cereal, candy, raw sugar, etc. A great time to utilize simple carbs is before, during, and right after training or practice. Consuming carbs then will help your body recover quicker and optimally.

Complex carbs (disaccharides) are a little more challenging for the body to break down. There is no rapid spike in blood sugar. The energy released is prolonged. These are your fruits, veggies, and grains. The complex carbs get broken down into simple carbs and then go through the absorption and utilization process. There is an extra step with complex carbs, which requires more time and work for the body. Yet the math is still the same: 1 gram of carbs = 4 calories.

One thing to note about protein and carbs in terms of post-workout recovery. Once you're done training, consume some carbs within twenty to thirty minutes. A drink like Gatorade works very well for your simple carbs. Then add a banana for a complex carbohydrates that is high on the glycemic index (the index that lists the sugar and macros for food items). After forty to fifty minutes of training, then add in your protein drink for muscle repair. Protein takes longer to process and slows down the digestive system. Therefore, get your sugar in first and get that traveling through your system with a short "head start." Then follow up with the slower protein source. Do *not* add in fat like peanut butter. Fat digests even slower than protein. This is by far the least effective macronutrient to add in this instance.

Let's look briefly at fiber before we analyze fats. Fiber is critical for your best bowel movements, lowering cholesterol, regulation of blood sugar, and better gut health. If you are struggling with your gut health, this is the first step in the process: Increase your fiber intake. You can do so by adding nuts, beans, cauliflower, green beans, potatoes, oats, apples, citrus fruits, and carrots. For further improved gut health add in cabbage and/or sauerkraut. Both will help tremendously.

Fats

Starting with the math, 1 gram of fat = 9 calories. More than double the other two, isn't it? This is the densest macronutrient and consequently the slowest for the body to process. Fat usually has a negative connotation. However, like the other two, fat is critical for the body to perform optimally. It provides energy reserves. It also provides satiety, which is feeling "full" after eating. Fat helps reduce inflammation, which is prevalent after training and practice/games. There is the obvious insulation which is seen visibly. For some sports, professions, and other ways of life, excess insulation is very necessary. Fat also aids in the production of hormones while protecting vital organs. Fat transports vitamins and improves blood vessel function and intra-artery plaque. Fat clearly has its place and value.

What are some examples of where athletes would need a decent amount of fat? Years ago on his radio show, Colin Cowherd interviewed former NFL quarterback Trent Dilfer. As an NFL athlete, you'd think that a very lean, strong athlete would be best. Not necessarily. As a quarterback, he often is in a defenseless position. Then he gets "trucked" by a defensive lineman. Well, the muscle and fat on his body help protect his bones and organs against the ferocity of the tackle, so it pays to have some "extra pudding" around the middle.

In two completely different sports, swimming and water polo, there is a little extra fat carried here as well. Granted, not very much. Athletes here are in the water so much that a lot of energy is being spent constantly from simply being in the water. The body is trying to regulate its temperature against the water. Then you must add in the work required to compete in your sport. Fat becomes a requirement here as well.

You'll find fat in most meats, nuts, but also some fruits and vegetables. When consuming a food item, be careful in how you categorize it. An item could have a high concentration of fat while you believe it's mostly protein, such as nuts, eggs, and peanut butter. Most will say they're a great source of protein. Well, they're good, not great. In fact, there is so much fat present that it's better to think of those items as more of a fat than a protein. The same is true for salmon. Salmon has great amounts of protein in it, but it's also not very lean. There is as much fat found in salmon as there is in a greasy cheeseburger. Other whitefish options have a much better ratio of fat to protein.

Let's look at omegas briefly. Omega-3 fats are a key family of polyunsaturated fats. Omega-3s have been shown to help prevent heart disease and stroke, may affect lupus and arthritis, and may play a role in cancer and other conditions. Omega-6 is also a polyunsaturated fatty acid. Omega-6s play a crucial role in brain function and normal growth and development as well as stimulating skin and hair growth, supporting bone health, regulating metabolism, and supporting the reproductive system. Clearly, 3s and 6s have value. The issue becomes what is a good ratio of 3s to 6s? The answer is one to four of 3s to 6s. Omega-3s are found in salmon, tuna, flaxseed, and chia seeds. Omega-6s are found in other nuts, seeds, and vegetable oils. Process? Track your intake for one to two weeks and find the math of your 3s versus your 6s. Then rebalance your food intake to optimize your omega ratio. Easier process? Take a high-quality omega supplement.

On a smaller scale, foods have micronutrients as well as macronutrients. Makes sense, right? Macros are larger, and micros are smaller, obviously. The macros are the higher priority, but micros provide enormous value as well. Micros are your vitamins and minerals. You can consume these via your food intake or through supplements (pills and powders). We'll get into them later. A simple rule here is eat fruits and vegetables at every meal and you'll hit 90 percent of your micros. Problem solved. Keep things simple and hit this habit, and you'll be just fine.

Remember, there is no perfect food. And you'll need a combination of the three macronutrients for you to perform as an athlete or simply to live. The next question becomes what do you need to eat? How much? How often? The answer is easy but requires more questions. In your sport, what is the level of athlete you're striving to become? Pretender? College Athlete? Pro? Or the Statue? What does he or she look like? What can he or she do physically? Then you must create your body to look and perform like the athlete you are becoming.

My son Jack left to play football for Ball State University in the summer of 2021. He weighed in at 207 lb. and was six-foot-one. He currently plays linebacker. When he left for school, he back squatted 500 lb., power cleaned 300 lb., and benched 300 lb. He ran in the 4.8 range in the forty-yard dash. In a lot of ways, he had very good numbers for someone right out of high school. His overall size was significantly smaller than required. And he needed to get quicker. I went through all the linebackers in his conference, the Mac. Then I went through the Big Ten as well. 90+ percent of the linebackers weighed between 220 lb. and 245 lb. They were roughly an inch to an inch and a half taller too (can't coach height). The next problem was that I couldn't find the physical measurables for the linebackers in the conference. I needed more data. I reached out to Ohio State's football program and asked if I could shadow them for a day with the strength and conditioning program. (Mickey Marotti and Quinn Barham were immensely helpful! Thank you!) I learned too many things in one day to list here. But here is something easy to find. OSU had the results listed on the wall for everyone within the top 10 percent and 25 percent for the most recent year's NFL draft, meaning the average five-ten-five drill, bench press numbers, vertical jump, broad jump, etc. are listed by position. Bingo! Then I got the information to Jack. His job was to train to get to that level if, and only if, his goal was to get to pro-level numbers. Once he developed his body and had the physical measurables, then he could confidently "check that box" for what it takes to be a pro-level athlete. This is what he needed to evolve to. There is clearly more to being an NFL player than that. But now he had the targets. From there, it's up to him to get there. And you can readily Google the info on the internet and find it for yourself as well. Will you be Disciplined and Relentless enough to get there? We'll see.

Bomb Shakes

Another real-life example: Most athletes are generally lean and trying to get bigger, faster, stronger. Not always. Some are overweight and need to lose body fat. Others need not be much bigger, like runners. It always depends. But some need an enormous number of calories to maintain their output or put on size to increase their output. Chad Dockery helped us out and introduced bomb shakes to Jack. It was what several football players, swimmers, and other athletes would do to keep their calories high. Have one or at most two bomb shakes each day until you are at the body composition you must have to dominate. Put everything in the shake but the kitchen sink. Here is what you're looking for:

- 60 g of protein.
- Whole milk and ice cream.
- Any other "junk" you like for more calories.
- Your creatine supplement.
- Peanut butter or other fats.
- Goal: 1,500+ calories per shake.

Jack and Sam would put in Oreos, chocolate syrup, pancake syrup, cereal, or anything he wanted. Some guys would put in raw eggs for the fat content. The point isn't to be healthy with great, whole foods with this habit. The point is to give the body enough fuel for it to handle the workload. Think like this: Some marathoners are eating while running. Swimmers eat all day, every day, everything they want, and still lose weight and muscle mass. If you need a lot of fuel, it's impossible to eat 100 percent clean. You'll have to eat a little dirty. In the end, it takes what it takes. Find a way. Win.

CHAPTER 36

NUTRITION - WAY OF INCHES

Process is king. Let's look at, analyze, and improve your Nutrition process. Recall that the first step in looking at your eating habits is learning what you eat. You must find a starting point. It's time for the Nutrition portion of the self-assessment test. Focus solely on the Nutrition Block for this exercise.

The following is the Inches Way: Nutrition section of the Assessment Test

NUTRITION

Body Fat

- 10 Points: You are in the top 10 percent (in body fat) at your position nationwide.
- 8 Points: You are in the top 10 percent in your conference.
- 6 Points: You are in the top 10 percent of your position group on team.
- 4 Points: You are in the top 20 percent of your position group on the team.
- 2 Points: You are in the top 50 percent of your position group on the team.

- 0 Points: All else.

POINTS: _____

Protein, Creatine, and Supplements

- 10 Points: You have a process to perfect performance and adhere to it always.
- 8 Points: You mostly have a process and adhere to it.
- 6 Points: You sometimes have a process and adhere to it.
- 4 Points: You rarely have a process and adhere to it.
- 0 Points: All else.

POINTS: _____

Offseason Total Nutrition Plan

- 10 Points: You have a process to perfect performance and adhere to it always.
- 8 Points: You mostly have a process and adhere to it.
- 6 Points: You sometimes have a process and adhere to it.
- 4 Points: You rarely have a process and adhere to it.
- 0 Points: All else.

POINTS: _____

In-season Home Games

- 10 Points: You have a process to perfect performance and adhere to it always.
- 8 Points: You mostly have a process and adhere to it.
- 6 Points: You sometimes have a process and adhere to it.
- 4 Points: You rarely have a process and adhere to it.
- 0 Points: All else.

POINTS: _____

In-season Away Games

- 10 Points: You have a process to perfect performance and adhere to it always.
- 8 Points: You mostly have a process and adhere to it.
- 6 Points: You sometimes have a process and adhere to it.
- 4 Points: You rarely have a process and adhere to it.
- 0 Points: All else.

POINTS: _____

Kaizen

- 10 Points: You have a process for improving and adhere to it without fail.
- 8 Points: You mostly have a process and adhere to it.
- 5 Points: You occasionally have a process and adhere to it.
- 0 Points: All else.

POINTS: _____

Nutrition Mentor

- 10 Points: You have one and connect weekly.
- 8 Points: You have one and connect monthly.
- 5 Points: You have one and connect quarterly.
- 0 Points: All else.

POINTS: _____

How effectively are you working with a Nutrition accountability ally (or allies)?

- 10 Points: You and your ally review your results weekly, enforce a "carrot/stick," and adjust.
- 7 Points: You and your ally review your results monthly and sometimes enforce "carrot/stick."
- 4 Points: You and your ally review your results quarterly.
- 0 Points: All else.

POINTS: _____

You know your number one Nutrition Strength (Competitive Advantage):

- 10 points. Otherwise: 0 points.

POINTS: _____

You know your number one Nutrition Weakness (Weak Link):

- 10 points. Otherwise: 0 points.

POINTS: _____

You know your number one Nutrition Opportunity (Target):

- 10 points. Otherwise: 0 points.

POINTS: _____

You know your number one Nutrition Threat (Enemy):

- 10 points. Otherwise: 0 points.

POINTS: _____

TOTAL POINTS: _____

OVERALL AVERAGE (TOTAL POINTS /12) _____

You see your score. Retest yourself at the end of every quarter of the year (March 31, June 30, September 30, December 31).

Ask yourself a series of reflective questions and gauge your progress over the last quarter.

- What is your level of knowledge of how, when, and what to eat? Do you know the basics and have a general understanding of what it takes to eat well?
- What have your habits been? Can you quantify what's required to compete at a high level?
- Who has been a solid Nutrition Teammate and who has not?
- What are your next steps to level up your Kaizen approach to your Nutrition process?

SWOT analysis. This time, apply your SWOT analysis to the Nutrition Block. Be sure to prioritize and identify your Competitive Advantage and your Weak Link. You must advance in these areas to optimize your performance. Write out your process goals and habits for the next quarter. What is your number one target for this quarter? Share with your Nutrition accountability ally. Devise your carrot and stick for your check-ins. Bring on a mentor as well. I can't imagine a scenario where you work this diligently and don't advance. It's impossible. You'll continue to crush it.

- Strength:
  - List them all.
  - What are your top three?
  - What is your number one Strength (Competitive Advantage)?
- Weaknesses:
  - List them all.
  - What are your top three?
  - What is your number one Weakness (Weak Link)?
- Opportunities:
  - List them all.
  - What are your top three?
  - What is your number one Opportunity (Target)?
- Threats:
  - List them all.
  - What are your top three?
  - What is your number one Threat (Enemy)?

Nutrition Way of Inches

The improvement process is a bit different here than the other Inch Blocks thus far. Your Nutrition can be largely dependent on others and what's provided. Meaning, you may be subject to what's prepared for you at home and at school for what you eat. That's a fact. There is no need to complain or worry about it. You must adapt and overcome.

First you must communicate with your Teammates (those who prepare your food). If possible, make requests and see where the discussion leads you. It may get you nowhere. But it may also help "move the needle" and get you some more meats, fruits, and vegetables. Then you must work more on your own to fill in the gaps. You may need to work a little more to earn some money to get the food you need or the supplements you want. There is a difference between a walk-on athlete, a scholarship athlete, and an athlete with a NIL deal. The same is true in the pros. Remember, there is a solution to every problem.

Now work backward from where you want to be at the end of your career, college, and high school and this year, quarter, month, and week. Based on your answers above and your SWOT analysis, what is today's Inch Challenge? What days and times this week will you work on your Nutrition Inch Challenge?

What are the obstacles that get in the way? Identify them. These are the threats, your opponent, your enemy. Remember, you still need an Inch, so you need a solution to your obstacle.

At the end of your week, tally up your score. See how you did versus your plan. Give yourself the carrot or stick. And then revise your plan for next week. Wash, rinse, repeat. Attack, attack, attack. Win, win, win! Sustainability is the goal. Not one great day each month. Get a little bit better daily and build your Inch Blocks. See how much better you can build yourself, and your Inch building blocks will show it. Kaizen.

10 Nutrition Habits

Not sure where to start or feeling overwhelmed? Pick one at a time and make it a habit and then evolve it further. Here are the solid priorities for improving in the Nutrition area. Remember the push-ups and the Statue. Get there.

1. Get your baseline and figure out what you're eating. Use an app, your phone, OneNote, a notebook, or whatever works for you.

2. Calculate your protein number and design a process to hit that number daily. Roughly, consume 1 g of protein for 1 lb. of lean mass to maintain your body composition. Consume less than that ratio to lose weight and muscle. Consume more to gain size, muscle, and strength. How much more? Start with 20 percent more and see.

3. Calculate your calorie numbers and design a process to hit that number. You must see what you're eating currently and determine how many calories that is. Recall that you'll need an excess of about 3,500 calories to gain one pound of weight and a deficit of the same amount to lose one pound. Then plan to hit your calorie number daily. Once you have your protein and calorie number, you'll be fine with your fat and carbs. Remember, this is a basic approach.

4. Eat all the fruit and vegetables you can.

5. Drink enough water so that your urine is consistently a light lemonade color.

6. "Be not like dumb, driven cattle." Track your results and adjust week to week. Make one or two adjustments every two to four weeks. Do not add new habits until the current ones are ingrained into your identity. Eat to win.

7. Communicate your plans with your Teammates and accountability allies.

8. Take your five supplements: Vitamin D, probiotic, fish oil, creatine, and whey protein isolates. Set this purchase up on auto-ship to solidify your process.

9. Find someone to help you.

10. Teach your teammates so they improve. Then you'll have a better shot at winning.

<u>Scan the following QR code</u> or visit: https://athlete-builder.com to access and download the assessment in this chapter and other resources (free nutrition resources and free workout programs).

CHAPTER 37

RECOVERY

"It's not how hard you can train. It's how hard you can train, recover, and train as hard again, every day." – Jim Beebe

KISS: Keep It Simple Stupid (Navy SEAL directive). With that last sentence in mind, the top three "steroids" for you will be food, water, and sleep. If you maximize and optimize those three components, then you will cover the bulk of Recovery. Go back and reread the Nutrition section and make it happen. Eat the right foods in the right quantities. Take your main supplements. Drink a ton of water. And sleep as much as you can. You will be doing very well with Recovery.

Is that it, then? It depends. For some, the above paragraph will be such an enormous change that they could be set for over a year learning and working on those principles. Perhaps it will take even longer if starting at the bottom with their Recovery habits. For others, there is always a next step and progression. Hunt for it. Hunt weaknesses.

Not convinced? What's the first thing you want to do when you're sick? Probably sleep. How low is your energy to perform when you've skipped breakfast or other meals? Terrible. Ever stay up late studying, or more likely partying or on your phone? (For most, their phones are cancerous.) How do you feel the next day? Terrible. How much better do you feel getting a cold drink of water after competing in the sun all afternoon in July? Much better. You know it's true. You must improve your

Discipline with your Recovery process if you want to make it to the next level.

Still don't believe me? Stay up for forty-eight hours and then go to practice. See what happens. Now this example is extreme to illustrate a point. What's the more likely issue? It's this: You're sleep-deprived by thirty to ninety minutes every day for weeks, months, and years. You don't recognize that the little misses each night adding up. You falsely believe "well I just don't require that much sleep." This is pure ignorance and stupidity. As a growing athlete, trying to compete at his highest level, training his butt off, you're the magical unicorn snowflake that, while under all this stress of competing, doesn't need the minimum (let alone optimum) amount of sleep to perform at his best? Shut up. And take a nap.

The effect of not recovering is like boiling the frog. You don't realize it's happening until it's too late. This is how you shorten your career to not having one. Follow along here. Can we agree that sport is a game of Inches? If not, then you wasted your money on this book. Sport is a game of Inches. A few Inches off, and you either make the play or miss the play. What about this: You're sleep-deprived a little every day, or you're not recovering well, you'll play a little slower. Your reaction time is impacted, and now you're off by a few more Inches. Instead of missing the play by a few Inches, you're now off by six Inches, twelve Inches, etc. Obviously, that's worse. Here's the real kicker: When you're consistently out of position, you not only miss the play, but you increase the chance of injury! Why? Well, if you were operating optimally, you wouldn't have put yourself in that spot at that time to make the play. Now you're exposed. Your risk has increased. No one wants an injury. The setback could be career-ending depending on the severity of it.

Making it to the top takes everything. It also requires a little bit of luck. In the words of Louis Pasteur, "Fortune favors the prepared mind." Also, "Luck = Hard Work + Opportunity" –Bobby Knight. This means you create your own luck and minimize chance. Take as many of the matters in your own hands as possible. Neglect Recovery at your own peril. It's another critical Block you must build fully.

CHAPTER 38

RECOVERY - SLEEP

Yes, it's obvious that sleep is important. It's also simple to say, "Just go to sleep." However, optimizing your sleep is not so obvious. Luckily, we have some of the answers and the process for you. If there is one thing to focus on and maximize for your Recovery, it is unquestionably sleep. First, here is some of the basic information regarding sleep.

There are different stages of sleep:

- Stage 1: Lightest sleep. One to seven minutes. In the time-period right after you drift off from being awake.
- Stage 2: Light sleep. Ten to twenty-five minutes. Your body relaxes, and it's best to wake up during this stage.
- Stage 3: Deep sleep. Twenty to forty minutes. Your brain and body are recovering more during this stage. If you wake up now, you'll be groggy.
- Stage 4: Rapid Eye Movement (REM) sleep. This period is populated by vivid dreams and a feeling of unrest upon awakening.

Benefits of improved sleep include improved memory, reduced anxiety and depression, a boosted immune system, lowered risk of heart disease, healing of the body, and aided muscle growth and repair. Negatives of sleep deprivation include increased risk of Alzheimer's, increased levels of hormone Ghrelin causing hunger, 1.5 times higher likelihood of developing diabetes. If you average two hours of sleep less than needed, you are four times more likely of developing a cold and 27 percent more likely to experience a cardiovascular event.

Get more sleep! Get better sleep! Here's how:

- Schedule when you sleep and stick to it. Your body likes routines and habits and responds well to them. Establish a habit you can execute. If you are up late on the weekends but disciplined during the week, then you change your sleep pattern the same as traveling across the country every week. You create your own self-inflicted jet lag.
- Create your environment in your room and throughout where you live. This can be very hard if you share a room or have room-mates down the hall. Each person impacts the other. Teamwork is a Core Value.
  - Eliminate all light in your room, even from clocks, windows, etc. as best you can.
  - Have some "white noise" from a fan going in the background, sounds of the ocean from an app on your phone or anything else that has a constant, soothing hum to it.
  - Have your room as cold as possible. This helps your brain relax.
- Naps. Limit them if possible. You want to lengthen your time sleeping which will lengthen the Stage 3 and Stage 4 intervals. This provides the most recovery. However, if you can get in a long night session repeatedly and still add a nap, then by all means do it.
- Follow a champion's evening habits.
  - Don't drink much water in the late afternoons or early evening. You want to limit any trips to the bathroom.

- ◦ Limit caffeine intake in the afternoon and evening hours as well. The last thing you want is a stimulant close to bedtime.
- ◦ Limit your alcohol intake, too. Alcohol is essentially a poison that your body must work to process. You prefer that your body rest and not work while sleeping.
- ◦ Eliminate your screen time thirty to sixty minutes before sleeping. Scrolling on your phone, watching movies, and working on the computer all stimulate your brain. The light from the screens does this too. And if you're watching something with more stimulation (action, horror, tense shows), then your brain is on full alert. You're trying to get it to calm down so you can heal.
- ◦ Do something to calm yourself down before sleeping: mediation, prayer, journaling, or breathing techniques. Taking one of these steps helps you relax further and prepare your mind and body for what's next.
- Set multiple alarms away from your bed with multiple devices to insure no misses in the morning. I usually have champion-type songs linked to my alarms like the *Rocky* fight songs or the intro to Michael Jordan's home games with the Bulls. I also have directives written into the alarm settings: "Go out and attack today" or "Execute!"

A few of the methods mentioned here can be implemented immediately and easily. Others may take more time and effort. Like any habit, start small and gradually improve. You must have the habit before you improve the habit. Then reevaluate. Consistency is key. Process is king.

CHAPTER 39

RECOVERY - COLD THERAPY

W ithout a doubt, this is a love-hate aspect of Training and Recovery. Eventually it's simply what's next and part of the Way of Inches. There are two aspects to discuss here. First is the use of ice and cold therapy to help healing directly from training. Second is the aspect of using cold therapy for your overall health and wellness as well as Mindset training. Both are musts. You will need to add these two components as you climb to higher levels of your greatness.

Basic Healing

I'm sure at some point you've been hurt, sprained an ankle, or been hit in some fashion. Every athlete will have bumps and bruises, aches, and pains. Hopefully at this stage in your career you've been told to "put some ice on it" or had a part of your body wrapped in it. You may even have done an ice bath or two. I don't want to belabor the basics too much here. If you get banged up, see a trainer, or a doctor and they will most likely prescribe some sort of ice therapy for you. Or you'll simply apply it on your own as well. These are necessary, important steps. Do not take them lightly. Do it and get it done. Then you can move on to the next task.

Ice baths are the next step after more serious and severe training. It's rare that you'll see it in high school practices, but you could, depending on the level of sophistication at your school. Ice baths will be more prevalent, if not legislated, at the college and pro levels. In high school, both my sons, Jack and Sam, would do the basic lifting offered at their high school. Then they'd come to my gym so I could fix all the areas that were missed. Then they'd have practice. That is a lot of volume for a teenager. Consequently, we started doing basic ice baths in the family bathroom tub. Then we added in a large animal trough/outdoor tub for more practical ice baths. The second option was not very pretty. But both were very effective. It takes what it takes.

When your body is under a lot of duress, enormous inflammation occurs. Your body is trying to heal by sending red and white blood cells to the distressed areas. You'll feel like you're "running hot" for an extended period—because you are. Adding in an ice bath after hard practices or training sessions or after significant exposure to heat will go a long way toward your Recovery. Do not shy away from this. Jump in and do it. Fully immerse yourself up to your neck. That way, all areas of the body benefit. You'll want to remain there for two to five minutes. It is not fun, but it is necessary. It's best just to jump in and make it happen. Don't get in slowly, as it only makes matters worse. Also, do not "fight it." By that I mean do not tense up and internally fight against the stressor of the cold water. Simply take it in and breathe deeply. Relax. Go to a place in your head and remain calm through deep breathing. Let your body absorb the cold and utilize it.

Once you get out of the ice bath, you'll need to walk around and move about to help foster your circulation again. The blood will rush to the body's priorities first, helping the body heal. Like all habits, it'll get easier as you do it more often. With that said, this is one habit where your breath gets taken away each time you plunge in. That part doesn't seem to go away. Once you dry off, go about your day and onto the next task. You have more to do to be great.

Cold Therapy For Health, Wellness, and Mindset

I'm good at this. But Wim Hof is the expert in this area (www.wimhofmethod.com). His content is excellent. He has an app, and a website with courses, and great content on social media. If you look around the internet, there are a few Wim Hof certified instructors on his methods. I've been through one of the courses, and they are helpful. No question. And there is more to it than the cold therapy. Seek one out and attend. It's worth it.

Why do any form of cold therapy outside of recovering from training? There are several reasons. Like the reasons for training, once you exit the cold tub, your blood will rush to the troubled areas of your body with red and white blood cells. This facilitates healing again. The process of making your blood hot and cold helps improve your circulation as well. Some will alternate multiple times in a session from hot to cold to hot to cold again for this reason alone. Your aches and pains will subside from the cold therapy session. It helps with brain function and clarity as well. The repeated exposure to the cold will increase the body's level of brown fat. This "healthier" version of fat will work better at insulating the body from the elements. Essentially the body recognizes it will be exposed to the cold and will alter it as a form of protection.

You can take my word for it or not. You can look up the data and research it yourself or not. You may *feel* a certain way about it. You may *think* a certain way about it. Both how you feel and how you think are not relevant at all when compared to what you *know*. You must learn for yourself. Try it out and see. Do it for eight weeks and document it each time. What did you learn?

I can tell you I feel much better each time I finish it. I have more energy and am more alert the rest of the day afterward. I am rarely sick at all. It helps me calm down and reduce stress. That's the Mindset component. So many are terrified of even trying it. They "just can't." God, it makes me sick. Fear winning out. Disgusting. Take solace in the fact that you have the mental strength to handle a new challenge. Others won't, but you will. "Today I will do what others won't. Tomorrow I will do what others can't." – US Navy SEAL adage.

As of this writing, I'm eighteen months into doing some form of cold therapy every day. It works. My wife says that after two big knee surgeries, her knee feels the best after cold therapy. Two Highland games throwers do it daily in a great cold tub. Both the husband and wife say their normal levels of anxiety have been eliminated, and they are off their medications for anxiety. I sleep better while having more energy during the day. Try it out and see for yourself.

Process Is King

Here is how I started and still progress today. I began with a cold shower, not the tub. I would take a normal, hot shower. I'd wash everything and lather up. Then I'd rinse off. Next, I would turn the dial all the way to the cold, the water still coming out full force. From here, I would do the "hokey pokey." I looked at my watch and had a target of fifteen seconds. During the fifteen seconds, I would put my right arm in the water for a bit and then pull it out. Then I'd do the same with the left arm. That was it. Believe me. No other part of me was in the cold water! Mentally, I wasn't there yet. And fifteen seconds goes quickly. It's not much time at all. I repeated this daily for a week.

One week later, I continued the "hokey pokey" by adding another fifteen seconds for my legs. Now I was at thirty seconds total, and all in, it wasn't that bad. Another week went by, and I added fifteen seconds for my torso. You'll find your torso to be easier. It has more fat and muscle and therefore more blood. That part isn't hard at all. Now I was at just under a minute in three weeks. Progress.

When you turn around and the water hits your back, it stings a little bit. Every time. There is no getting around it. It just does. Add another fifteen seconds here and you hit your one-minute mark. That's great.

You'll find most of your benefits are realized when you get to two minutes consistently. Spend a minute on each side. That will be best.

Where am I at today? I do five minutes daily. And I don't bother with the hot water at all any longer. I was getting to the point that I was in the shower for ten minutes. It was taking too long, and I had things to do. The process now is no longer the "hokey pokey." I've learned something else. When I jump in now, I try to get all areas exposed as quickly as possible. Once my back gets hit with cold, then blood rushes to it, and it warms up. The same is true with all other areas. So I spend a minute turning around, getting all areas exposed, because I actually feel warmer in those areas for the duration of the shower. I make sure to spend the last minute with the water crashing into my face and the top of my head. Breathe through it. Don't fight things. Relax and accept it. You can handle it.

When it comes to the tub, follow a similar process. A few days prior to my Wim Hof course, I found myself getting a little nervous about the event. I had been doing cold showers for five months but no ice baths. Well, instead of waiting to find out how it would feel, I took matters into my own hands. I went and got a sixty-gallon tub and filled it with water. I threw in two large bags of ice and jumped in. The goal was two minutes, which I did. Then a week later, when I did the course, I knew I could handle it. It wasn't fun. But I survived. You will too. That day in February in Indiana, we were outside. The instructor filled this kiddie pool with water and dropped in a dozen large bags of ice. It was slushier than anything. He had us get in for ninety seconds. So, I went first because I like getting the hard tasks done immediately. It worked. I survived and was thrilled I completed it. Today I do the ice bath at least twice each week for five minutes. On days without the ice bath, I'm sure to get a cold shower in. To be clear, the shower is easier for me. On the other hand, my wife likes the ice bath better. The ice bath has a greater effect because you're fully submersed in it. With the shower, you can "hide" sometimes. Again, the best plan is the one you stick to. Either way, get in and get going. It's time to add in cold therapy to your routine.

CHAPTER 40

RECOVERY - BREATHING AND MEDITATION

Your mind and your body are miraculous things. It's truly amazing how you are already equipped to help yourself heal. Think for a moment and determine if I'm right or not. The speed at which injuries and illnesses can cure themselves is staggering. Once you add in professional help, you'll realize that your body will literally go wherever your mind dictates. Fact.

Let's address one of the fundamental methods for healing yourself: breathing. I'm sure we can agree that stress can be a significant challenge for the mind and the body. And the phrase "Calm down and take a breath" is timeless. Why? Obvious. You can impact your mind and body with your breathing. Then you must use it to your benefit.

How? Breathing techniques affect the body's biochemistry. It affects how the electric impulses flow in the nervous system. This process makes the body more alkaline, which enables the electric impulses to flow more freely and quickly. Your muscles, controlled by the brain, are governed by these electric impulses. Breathing deeply increases the amount of oxygen into the body. Now more oxygen is traveling to areas that typically receive less because of the constant shallow breathing. This increased oxygen makes the body more alkaline, improves the electric impulses flowing, improves brain and muscle function, and therefore improves performance. Your muscles perform better. Your reaction time is better. You think more clearly. You can focus even better.

Lamaze

Millions of expectant mothers have taken a Lamaze class in preparation for delivering a baby. There are a few components to the approach. However, the main tactic is breathing because it helps calm the body and mind. The basic breathing approach is:

1. Sit upright. Breathe in slowly and deeply through your nose filling your lungs fully. Use your diaphragm as much as possible. Do this within four seconds.
2. Hold your breath for four seconds.
3. Exhale fully taking four seconds.
4. Hold your breath again for four seconds.
5. Continue repeatedly. Do ten rounds. Then work your way up to three to five minutes.

The process enables the mother to handle the significant pain that ensues. It also helps her calm down. It will lower her heart rate, which is under constant duress during the process. Now that she is more in command of her mind and body, she can focus much better. Each benefit feeds the other benefit and helps you survive and manage the process.

Box Breathing

Mark Divine, a retired Navy SEAL and head of SEALFit, did not invent box breathing. It's a common technique he and all military branches teach. Although Mark didn't invent it, he certainly is wise enough to utilize it and teach it to anyone who will listen. What is the box breathing method? Good question. Answer: It's the exact same method as Lamaze, just with a different name. Why or when would

Mark and others utilize the method? There are too many answers to list them all. A few examples:

- It's done prior to training to help the athletes, soldiers/sailors, marines, etc. focus.
- It's done prior to a stressful conflict (e.g., going into battle, going into a close-quarters conflict, or any other physical altercation).
- It's done by snipers to help them calm down and focus on the targets.

Childbirth and military combat are life-and-death situations. In both cases, employing some breathing techniques and habits will make all the difference. The methods have been taught for more than a half century for both groups. We would be foolish to ignore the knowledge and not benefit from its practice. Therefore, we must take advantage of the techniques and gain another Inch. It's a tool in your belt that will improve your performance. And that's what we are after.

Wim Hof's Method

Hof and his coaches teach a method that helps people deal with stress and lower their overall stress levels. The method is much more involved and takes a bit longer to perform. But the ability to relieve stress has been great. The process is this:

1. Start first thing in the morning.
2. Lie down flat on the floor on your back.
3. Breathe in deeply and fully. Fill "your belly" first and through the "top of your lungs." Do this as quickly as possible.
4. Then breathe out fully and as quickly as possible.
5. Repeat thirty to forty times.
6. Take in one more deep breath and let out about half the air.

7. Hold it and time yourself. Hold it as long as you can without significant discomfort.
8. Then inhale once more and hold for about fifteen seconds.
9. Repeat this process again.
10. When it's time to hold your breath again, invariably it will happen naturally for much longer.
11. Repeat the process for a third time.
12. The third time you hold your breath will be the longest you're able to hold it.
13. Repeat this habit daily.
14. Track your results and assess for yourself.

It'll help clear your head. It will also give you a chance to think and focus on what you must accomplish that day. In addition, there are the mental benefits for reduced stress levels. Keep notes in your journal to see how you progress.

Game Day and Making a Play

What about in the moment? Or what about right after the moment when the next moment is coming at you quickly? It depends. It really depends on your sport. I can't think of any sports where you can lie down on the floor or the turf and go through the Wim Hof process. It's not likely you can stop and complete one minute of box breathing either. So, what can you do?

- You can do your Wim Hof breathing first thing in the morning.
- You can do some box breathing in the locker room prior to the game starting.
- You can do a few bouts of box breathing when you're resting on the bench after playing.
- **Key Moment:** If you have a moment or stoppage in play (about to perform a free throw in basketball, in the huddle in football

or time out, stepping into the batter's box or about the step on the pitching mound rubber, etc.) take one, two, or three deep breaths. Be deliberate. Do this consistently. In each instance you must have a predetermined mantra. The breathing will calm you. The mantra will direct your actions and focus. Now execute Relentlessly. Repeat the process.

It's okay to be an emotional player. It's okay to "play angry". It's not okay to be reckless and out of control. Being able to control yourself is paramount to winning. So, get fired up; get pissed off if you want to. But harness that and unleash it when the opportunity presents itself. Your breathing will help you remain in charge of your feelings, especially when you find yourself starting to boil over. Then make the opposition regret ever testing you. Take your abilities to a new level. Then continue to build and win.

One other thing that is helpful is calming yourself in preparation for sleeping. Recall in the Recovery section that optimizing your sleep helps you recover fully. Since that's the case, take five minutes prior to sleeping and center yourself again. Do five minutes of box breathing. Recall a reason to be grateful during this time. Or use it to meditate on something else. Prayer is extremely beneficial as well. Then when you turn in for the night, your mind and body already have a head start on the Recovery process. Get another Inch here if you can.

Directing Your Mind

The real, significant challenge is to calm your mind down. It can take weeks and months to get to the point where you can sit and "be still" in your thoughts for five minutes. Give it a try and see for yourself. You'll find your mind jumping from thought to thought. Even as you improve at directing your mind to "go blank," you'll still slip, and thoughts will creep in. It happens.

What do we do when that occurs? First, simply note what thoughts arise. It could be useless and meaningless. Or it could be a priority or issue you should address today. Either way, the task now is to train your mind to be still. When a thought enters my mind, I envision that I'm inhaling my thought in through my nose. And then I exhale the thought out of my mouth. In my mind, the thought leaves my mouth sealed up inside a clear plastic bag. And the thought floats away. I'll find my thoughts later, when I'm done with the exercise, if I want to.

This is a valuable exercise. You may want to add in a slight hum or *ohm* sound as you're meditating. Or not. It's up to you. Simply sit up straight on the floor and set your timer and be still. This is a fantastic exercise done in the morning to set your mood for the day. It's great prior to bedtime to help you relax and sleep better. You can also implement it after a stressful event if you have a moment. Being able to calm yourself amid a storm of stress will help you handle the stress in the first place. Ray Dalio, the founder of Bridgewater (one of the largest investment firms in the history of the world) was asked what some of his most valuable habits are. He immediately responded that his best one is to mediate one or two times each day for twenty minutes. He said it helped calm him and manage his thoughts from the day. It also helped his mind break down and process events and create new ideas.

Calming yourself has tremendous benefits. Directing your thoughts allows your mind to advance to a whole new level. Here's how. Just prior to doing your breathing and meditating, think about a phrase or mantra you must implement today. What are some big events or challenges you'll face? How must you handle and respond to them? Then come up with a word or phrase that encapsulates how you must handle those situations. Next set your breathing/meditation time for five minutes. Use the first three minutes to go through the process of calming yourself. Calm your breathing and do it deliberately. Eliminate thoughts in your mind. Let your thoughts float away for another time. Then at the three-minute mark, continue the process with your breathing. However, for the remaining time, focus intently on the mantra or phrase you'll need to guide you today. It could be a directive, a prayer, or a Mindset. This phrase will be your theme today. It's one that you want to shape your thoughts and actions. Direct and train your mind to be a force that helps you accomplish the tasks laid before you today. Then go out and execute like you can.

I usually like one-word mantras. Often, it's simply "Execute." Once I'm done with the breathing and clearing my mind, my overarching thought is to execute today. Get my tasks done. Work through my processes. Do the hard projects well and now. Other times I may have a series of contentious meetings scheduled. Even though I know that conflict is valuable and the best chance to grow, I don't often look forward to conflict with people. I don't avoid the conflict, but I try to run to it and address it before it festers and escalates. When I have a day like that, the mantra I select is "Peace." I want to remain calm during the conflict so my mind can be as logical as possible. I want to make the best decisions and statements to advance and improve from the situations.

As a physical example, squat day is the best day of the week in the gym. When I know it's squat day, I know that all my faculties must be on point for me to perform. It's especially true when I'm attempting a new max weight, or a max rep set. You really need to be dialed in and focused. Your best bet is to prepare Relentlessly all the other days, so that the day you max out is a forgone conclusion. Sun Tzu: "All battles are won before they are ever fought." Still, after training well leading up to today's challenge, you must focus and execute. My meditation mantra then would be "Drive and Aggressive." I want to drive my entire body into the bar and aggressively push it up. It's a singular focus on the task at hand. All concentration is directed and winning the challenge and standing up with the weight.

One time we were maxing out our back squat. It was 2014 and Dustin Burford was training me. I'm about to hit as many reps as possible with 405 lb. on my back. My kids were in the gym just screwing around while we were training. Dustin goes over and asks my daughter, Maddie, to come sit in front of my squat rack while I hit this set. In that instance, my thoughts just prior to it were "For Maddie, for Maddie, for Maddie." Over and over and over again. Each rep was increasingly painful but, in my mind, it was for my daughter. "Don't give up. Don't quit on this rep. Get another one. Go again. Go again! Go *again*!" Dustin was a great training partner. As the lifter, you must put your trust in your partners because your mind will play tricks on you and try to negotiate its way out of pain. Dustin was tasked with determining when my last rep would be based on my form and speed. After eleven reps, he had me rack the weight, and I sat down on a bench to recover. A set like that isn't done often. It's a nervous system wrecker. But I was able to "go to that dark place" and execute. I had a "Why:" for my daughter. It was my focus and directive. Then I simply and painfully would "go all in." Do the best I could in that moment. You learn a lot about what that feels like. You learn you can go to places mentally and perform. Confidence improves. You'll improve physically too from efforts like that. It's tremendous.

Another example: Jack was going into a typical football practice at Ball State. He wanted to make sure he was in the right position on each play. He also wanted to be there as fast as he could get there. Once he was in position to make a play or be in contact, he wanted to be as physical as possible. In this instance, the mantra is easy. It's "fast and physical." Get to the point of contact and hit whatever is in your way with everything you have. Bring the ball carrier down. Or knock all the blockers into the ball carrier. Knock the ball loose and get it. Win.

Using your breathing and mantra to direct your mind can be a powerful weapon. Train it like you train anything else. See what this tool can do for you.

CHAPTER 41

RECOVERY - TRAINERS AND DOCS

I t still "takes a village" to make the best athlete you'll ever be. You must use all resources. You must leverage other people's knowledge and experience. What does that mean? You must take what others know and can do and use it to your benefit. Basic example: You go to the dentist so he or she can clean and fix your teeth. You can only do so much alone. The experts in other areas must help you. The same is true with your Training and Recovery.

At the high school, college, and pro level you'll have some professionals on staff to help you recover. Use them as much as possible. Get as much from them as you can. When you're younger and not banged up, you may not feel the need to see them. (Reminder: Your feelings are useless.) What do you know? Answer: zero or very little. See them anyway. Get worked on. And learn! At some point, you'll really need some help and knowledge, and the trainer or doc might not be around right then. Learn how to foam roll, deeply massage yourself, use voodoo floss, and increase your range or motion, flexibility, and mobility. If you don't know these things, you need to. Kelly Starrett's online service is pure gold: www.thereadystate.com. Learn to love what is put out here.

Ask the trainers/docs all the questions you can. Take notes. Be an athlete. Be a professional. Question what they are doing as well. The absolute dumbest person to graduate from medical school is still called a doctor. There is no way that a new doctor fresh out of school will have the knowledge that a thirty-year seasoned veteran will have. Always ask questions to learn more.

Seek the experts in the field. Do not settle here. You're trying to be the Statue-level athlete. Seek out the Statue-level experts. Here are two real life examples:

My wife was competing at the Highlander Nationals in her age class in Ohio. A Highlander event is a combination of Highland games and strongman. She won the whole thing. Cool, right? Yes, it is. She won the last event, log press, as well, but she also blew out her knee on it. Not cool. We made it back to Indiana. The next day she needed to find a knee doctor. She could find one in her network, out of network, a specialist, or a general orthopedic doctor (a doctor who works on different bones and joints). She sought out "the man:" Dr. Klootwyk at Methodist Sports Medicine. This guy is up there in years. He only does knees. He's the knee surgeon for the Indianapolis Colts and Indiana State University football teams. His halls are covered with pictures of pro athletes he fixed up. She went to him. His entire staff is a finely tuned machine. Each employee overservices the patient. And Dr. K. is the true expert in his field. If you get injured, find the best like him.

Another example: Jack broke his back training at his high school his sophomore year. The spine doctor was a bit younger and worked on the entire body for athletes. He was a fine doctor, but Jack was failing to recover and heal. He needed to progress to get back in the game. I started asking around the local medical experts for a referral. They all pointed me to Andy Smith with Community Health Network. He was a sixty-minute drive one way, but he was worth it. His treatments were good. But the homework he had Jack do was critical. Jack was doing his exercises five times a day and healed up quickly. Smith only works on spines and has been doing it his whole life. Problem solved. Jack healed up in time for summer football. He was horribly weak and out of shape. How weak? He couldn't do one legit push-up. Once he received the green light, I trained him back up. He was a week-one starter. By the end of the season, he was playing both ways in football.

What if you're not optimizing your recovery with the resources you have? This happens. It's okay. We will come up with a plan to advance beyond it. First, take the free treatments and what's given to you as a player. Maximize those first. Then if you need more, get more. Meaning, if you need a chiropractor, which you do, then seek out one. Find one who works with athletes. More specifically find one who is well-versed in the Stuart McGill methods. (You can find some valuable resources and books by Stuart McGill on Amazon.) If you need dry needling or cupping, then find someone who does it. James Harrison, the legendary Pittsburgh Steeler would pay $300–400,000 a year on recovery. Take that same approach. Maybe you don't have that kind of money, but you can earn enough money to cover the cost of a chiropractor, so your body is aligned and running optimally. If you're in the Indianapolis area, find chiropractor Dr. Josh Healy in Mooresville. If you need a trainer, find Sara Hemmick Richardson with Myo-Fit, www.myofittherapy.com. Or consult the "Strongman Doc" Dr. Todd McDougle www.drmcdougle.com.

Don't have any money? Then it's the DIY route. Is this optimal? Nope. Is it the best right now? Darn right. So, you do what you can and move forward. Get some books or watch some YouTube videos. I put out content all the time, so you can learn new tips and tricks there. Either way, if you can't utilize an expert, then you must become the resident mini-expert. There is nothing wrong with that. Even the best doesn't have a team of doctors and trainers following them around every second of the day. You must do some work yourself. So, just do it.

CHAPTER 42

RECOVERY - MUSIC

M usic for recovery? Really? Of course it is. If you ever get a massage, you'll typically hear some soothing music playing. Why? It can have a calming effect. On the other hand, some music clearly can have the opposite effect as well. If you're listening to something soft and light versus something hard and fast, then you will impact your mind and body.

First, let's look at the stimulus aspect briefly. After all, this section is on Recovery. Recall the Brainwashing section earlier in the book. On your way to practice or a game, you can listen to something motivational, such as motivational music, to help prepare you for the challenges of the day. You'll often, if not daily, have aggressive music blaring in the weight room as you train. The loudspeakers are going full tilt during the game. There is even the school band playing trying to incite and stimulate the crowd. This in turn stimulates the athlete. This point is obvious and doesn't need to be belabored. It just is the way it is.

But think for a moment. Can you train a little differently regarding music? Should you even consider it? Let's first ask, is your music for training being used as a stimulant? Most likely, it is. It's very likely the entire point of it. Well, do people build up a tolerance to stimulants? Yes, they sure do. Now what? Answer: Cut out all music occasionally. Get "in your head" and train. Train like a savage, with only your thoughts to guide you. See where your mind wanders to and push. Zydrunas Savickas from Lithuania is regarded as one the best strongman competitors in the history of the sport, if not the best. When he trains, there is never music. It is simply him and his training partners getting after it. That's it. Then when he's onstage competing, there is plenty of music. There is also the crowd, the lights, the effects. Everything. It's a ton of stimulus. When interviewed, he was asked why there was no music. Simple. He wanted to lower his conditioning to the stimuli. Then when the moment counts, all the effects can elevate his mind and consequently his body. It's a method he employs. Give it a shot a few times and see. Try it for a month. You'll learn some more about you.

As for Recovery, you can use music or sounds several different ways. At this moment, you're looking to bring yourself from an elevated, hyper state down to a calmer more relaxed state. Have a playlist or set of songs and sounds to do so.

Gym example: It's a time of constant conflict within the gym as a coach and as an athlete. As an athlete, it's me versus the bar. It's me versus the task (sets and reps) and the pain. It's your Teammates pushing you and each other. It's the music pushing you, too. As a coach, it's some of the same issues. But it can also be me versus the athlete. It's my mind versus his mind. He may think he can't get the next set. But based on what I've seen, I know if he can or not. Now I must connect with the athlete and get him to trust me. I must get him to believe in my words and himself. I ask; he gives. It takes enough new, incremental conflict for an athlete's mind and body to evolve and adapt.

Now it's the end of the day. I'm done training. I'm done pushing athletes. I'm done pushing all my coaches to perform. I must drive ten minutes home and not walk through the door like a raging lunatic. And sometimes I am that lunatic when I get home. I need to detox and destress. What do I listen to so I can calm down? Usually just jazz music at night. If I have any hope of falling asleep or unwinding at all, I must start the process immediately. I might as well start as soon as possible on the ride home. On one hand, we use music in the gym or before a practice or game as a stimulant to get us pumped up. On the other hand, we use music to calm down and decompress. It's simply another tool to use for help throughout the day. Since that's the case, be deliberate about it. And maximize the benefits.

Side note: For a 1RM (one-rep max) lift, my go to are "The Haka" performed by New Zealand's rugby team, "Bawitdaba" by Kid Rock, "Bullets" by Creed, anything from the *Rocky* soundtracks, and a few others.

We already mentioned having some "white noise" in the background to help you sleep. This static noise or "song" has a calming effect. You can also use sounds of nature like running water, waves in the ocean, rain, etc.

I also like to listen to chants when I'm in the ice bath or when I'm doing my breathing and meditation. I'll find sounds of Tibetan monks chanting or Gregorian monks chanting. It helps calm me and center me.

The point is this: There are times when you need to be in an elevated state. Other times, you need a relaxed state. Use music as another tool to help with each. But don't forget to eliminate the music altogether and see where your mind goes. Learn from each experience and see what works for you at different times. Then apply and execute when you must. Get another Inch and win.

CHAPTER 43

RECOVERY - FLIPPING THE SWITCH

In the Mindset section, we looked at "flipping the switch" as you're about to focus fully on your next competitive task. It could be a big lift in the gym. Or it could be when you take the court, field, or ice for your sport. It could be as you're about to fight on the street. It's the Mindset switch where you go "all in" against your opponent. All hesitation and restraint are gone. In the fight or flight mentality, in this instance it is clearly a fight!

This scenario has nothing to do with Recovery. There is a plethora of times where you must at once change your Mindset quickly as your situation and circumstances change. Say that you just finished your 6:00 a.m. workouts in college. You shower up. Then you're off to an English class to discuss writing essays. That class is not the place for you to be overhyped, loud, and aggressive. It happens at work. It happens at home with the family. It happens with friends. An event occurs. You immediately feel an emotional response. What transpires next is the outcome. Make no mistake. It is *not* the event. It's how you responded to the event. You know it's true. You know it's right.

In fact, at this point in my life, I have so many things going on that I experience constant wins and losses all day every day. There is always some idiot in my life saying and doing things that could impact me. There is no shortage of stupid everywhere. You and I are surrounded by people's screw-ups that affect what we are trying to do. It happens all the time. And at forty-eight years old, I'm aware enough that I am often at fault as well, with too many of my own screw-ups to count. That's just life. There will never be a shortage of obstacles. And thank Jesus for them. You must be able to handle the small obstacles to prepare you for the large ones. And the large ones prepare you for the life-altering obstacles. God won't give you anything you can't handle.

Let's look at three steps to take when something (typically negative but sometimes positive) occurs. And your next response is critical in determining the outcome. Break down the next steps mechanically and logically. Put yourself in a detached mindset and find the best route forward. Ridiculously easy example: You walk into a room to get some studying done. You want to be able to study. Obviously, the obstacle is darkness. Your reaction is to turn on the light switch. Problem solved.

Here is why I like this example. I compare the light switch event to walking from one room to another. If it matters what's in the next room (like if I come home from training and my family is in the next room for dinner), then the first thing I want to do is determine the intent I must have to perform well in the next room. In this case, it's the next situation. What is the outcome I want? If I remember the outcome I want, then I can look critically at the event or obstacle before me. It makes it easier to go into problem-solving mode and execute. Too many times in my life I would go into pissed-off raging lunatic Jim Beebe mode. The outcome never really went well after that point. You must have a strong intention of how you want to work when you walk into the weight room, or into the team room for a discussion, or onto the playing field or court. The point is to be intentional and deliberate. Focus. Execute.

The next step is a calming method we already looked at earlier. Take a breath. As a kid I would hear, "take ten deep breaths, Jimmy, before you do anything." Or I would be told to count to ten aloud and slowly. Man, is that step annoying. Instinctively I want to fly off the handle and starting raging at people. Again, being young and immature has its drawbacks. This step in the process is critical. It slows the moment down and gives your mind a chance to override its feelings. Then it can operate optimally and give you a chance to win.

The third step is mechanical. Focus only on the next step and solve the problem. Win. To summarize, you have an event before you. You take a moment to remind yourself what your intent is with this event. The event occurs, and instinct and emotions kick in. You take a moment to calm yourself and center yourself back to a state of control. And the last piece is handling the event as best you can. Keep your intent in mind. It will help guide you through the process. The following are some examples for you to apply this process of Recovery.

Coaching example: I spent the last three hours coaching nonstop. It's constant aggression trying to get other coaches to perform optimally. And the same is true for the athletes. I get in the car to head home for the evening. What happens next will determine how well my evening goes. My intent is obvious: Enjoy dinner and the conversations with my family members. Head to bed in a relaxed state. Allow myself to start fresh the next day. The situation and obstacle are that I'm still jacked up for the prior several hours. It's late, another endless twelve- to fourteen-hour day. I'm hungry and in an aggressive mood. To help break the mindset and recover, I will either listen to some easy or calming music. Or I may listen to nothing at all and just try to relax. Depending on the weather, I might set up my Jeep with the top off to enjoy it. Once I pull into the garage, I'll sit there for twenty seconds, breathe deeply, and find gratitude. Most likely, I'm very thankful that food was prepared for me. It's a chore I didn't make time for, so it really helps me. Then I think about something fun to discuss with my wife or kids and let the evening unfold. It really helps a lot. Now, to be clear, I don't do this every time. I'll forget my Discipline and underperform. But at least I have and know a process. Then the more I execute it, the better I feel and do.

How does the above example apply to you? You have a hard day at school and practice. You're tired and pissed off. You come home and let your emotions control you. If you live at home with your family, that next moment won't go well. Your evening will continue to worsen. If you have roommates, there is a good chance they'll see how you are and start to mess with you. Either way, the prior events are now in control of your current mood. You are too weak to handle it emotionally. The event controls you. You continue to lose. That sucks. Stop the insanity and break the cycle.

Game day: Your intent is to win the game. Your intent is to win the next play. The entire game consists of ups and downs, obstacles, and adversity. Mistakes occur. Bad plays happen. The refs make the wrong calls. Some players cheat. Another player tries to injure you. The crowd is getting in your head. You worry about getting benched. You worry about this and that. None of that matters. Your only concern is the next play. Broken down further, your only concern is your next step forward. There's a break in the action. It's a time out, a penalty, or an injury stoppage. Remember, what is your intent? What is your mantra for the day? If it's "fast and physical," then your intent is to win by playing fast and physical. You are now given a gift: The game stopped. Breathe! Calm down. Look around. Assess what's about to happen next. Decide. Commit. Execute your mantra Relentlessly. This is the only way to affect the next step and the outcome.

As an exercise, scrutinize each factor I listed above. Write out how each one changes your mind and your body. Yes, there will be impacts on both. But do either of those factors control your mind and body? If you answer yes, then you agree that someone or something else controls you. You are no longer the boss of you. Taken a step further, if that's true and you're not in charge, then you are clearly too weak to win. You are too weak to advance. You don't have it right now. Until you can learn how to recover and take control of your mind and body, you will grossly underperform. This issue must be reconditioned and fixed. And make no mistake: This habit and process will challenge you repeatedly at different levels in your career. The process is the process. It's just how well you can execute your process.

Another example: You have a great practice. The coach is loving on you. You leave the practice facility jacked up. Now it's time to sit down in class and take a test. But you're still riding high, staring out the window thinking about how well you did. But the task at hand is the test. You need to recover from the positive experience to focus on the test. All that matters is the next step. Get back your Discipline and execute.

Another example: Your coach has been riding you all week long. And the last practice he was all over you, and tomorrow is the big rivalry game. You stop by her office to talk about your play. Can you see where I'm going with this? You must have an intention as you walk into her office. You have a desired outcome. How will you play your role in the next ten-minute meeting? What's your mantra? Can you be humble and vulnerable? If so, then you can hear and learn clearly what you must do to perform better. If your feelings are hurt and you can't hear the message, then you can't apply anything. You are unable to improve. You must be stronger than your feelings. You are looking for Knowledge from your coach on how to play better. That's the intent. That's the desired outcome. Everyone makes mistakes, and coaches know that. But if you can teach your coach that you immediately correct your mistakes, then she will give you more feedback and data. Then you can correct and improve your game even quicker. She will learn that you are the best at improving because you take in all her Knowledge faster and better than anyone else. Your advance rate is the best because you learn and apply everything the fastest. Adopt this approach to advance faster than your competitors.

CHAPTER 44

RECOVERY - THE GIFT OF INJURY

This can be a hard one, especially if you let it. Injury = Time off. Time off = Setbacks. Right? Well, it depends.

Yes:

- You are not playing.
- You are not practicing.
- Muscle can weaken and atrophy.
- Speed can decrease.
- Flexibility and mobility can decrease.
- The person taking your place could do well and excel.
- Your team could underperform without you.
- Negative feelings could impact your mood.

No: Let's look at each "negative" listed above and see how a constructive reaction will impact the outcome positively for you and your team.

Not Playing or Practicing

Your injury has the time to heal. The rest of your body has time to heal. Your nervous system can recover as well.

Own it 100 percent. There was at least one reason you got injured. Figure out why so it's not repeated. As you're watching others get injured, figure out why they did. Then be sure not to repeat their mistakes as well. Example: You're weak. That's why you broke your collarbone. Answer: Commit to your Training to get stronger! Another example: You were out of position and got blindsided. Answer: Watch more film so your level of Knowledge increases.

You can watch your team practice more. You can watch your team compete. You can watch your opponents compete. On the surface, it sucks. I get it. But now you have plenty of hours to learn from others' success and mistakes. Absorb it all. Talk with coaches and Teammates more and learn constantly.

You can still work on your Training. There is some part of you that can move. It is not a time to give up. It is a time to address every area that's been neglected. Perhaps you didn't prioritize your mobility because of limited time. Well, make that happen now while you can. Either way, get your ass in the gym, figure out what you can do, and execute.

Watch a ton more film. You already weren't watching enough. Fact. Now take advantage and pump as much Knowledge and film into that as you can.

Getting Weaker and Slower in Some Areas

Get stronger and faster in other areas. Tore an ACL? Then smash your core, back, and upper body. Get stronger in your upper body. Get faster too. Broken collarbone? Strengthen your core, low back, and lower body. Lunge until your butt falls off. If one area will get weaker and atrophy and you use that as an excuse to let your entire body weaken and atrophy, then you don't have it at all.

If your coach can't help you train around your injury, then you must still figure it out. It takes what it takes. You must find someone who can help you. There is always a next step. If you don't believe that, then you don't have it at all.

Flexibility and Mobility Decrease

It will be true for the injured area. This is no excuse for the uninjured areas. At a minimum, build those areas up. At a maximum, improve the uninjured areas to a level surpassing their best levels and ranges of motion.

Read Dr. Kelly Starrett's *The Supple Leopard* and *Becoming a Supple Leopard*. Both are gold for athletes and their mobility and flexibility. Now you can apply the increased Knowledge here for the rest of your playing career and beyond.

Also read *The Gift of Injury* by Brian Carroll and Dr. Stuart McGill. Read this especially if you have back issues. I've had bulging, herniated discs for years. I also have severe stenosis in my spine. After reading this book, I learned what an expert McGill is as a chiropractor. Then I knew to seek out a chiropractor that utilizes McGill's methods. I found Dr. Josh Healy in Mooresville, Indiana. Long story short, in 2020 I really hurt my back badly again. At the time, my back surgeon wanted to schedule me for surgery. Healy worked on me, gave me homework and exercises, and I didn't end up needing surgery. Back surgery is one of the last things you'll ever want. Avoid it at all costs. But without the Knowledge of the doctors employing the McGill method, I wouldn't have known to look around for one. Knowledge is power. Process is king.

Someone Else Has Your Job on the Team. The Team is Impacted by Your Lack of Play.

Teamwork is a Core Value. Get your replacement better! Don't be afraid and insecure. Attack and move forward. Your job is to help the team win in any fashion. Make your replacement better.

Let's use a rating system to illustrate a point. Let's say a Statue-level player is at 100, a pro is at 90, a college athlete is at 80, high school 70, and so on below. Right now, you "grade out" as 85 at the college level. Your replacement is new and at an 80. Your job is to build him up to get to his best, maybe 83, 85, 88 or whatever. Just get him there. Here's the big question: Were you planning to remain at 85? Or were you planning to hit 89, 93, 99 or whatever? Good! The point is that your targets are further up the scale. So don't be weak and insecure that someone is trying to reach where you are currently. By the time they arrive, you'll be long gone on to bigger and better things.

Attitude and momentum are contagious. When one or two guys are supportive on the team, others join in. The strength of the pack is the wolf. And the strength of the wolf is the pack. The support roles are critical to the team's success. You need support when you're a starter. You must give it when you are not the starter.

Take extensive notes on your opponent's play. There is a good chance you will see this team, coach, or players again at some point. Watch and learn their tendencies, strengths, and weaknesses. Then use it against them later.

Negative Feelings Could Impact Your Mood.

This is true daily, whether you're injured or not. So, who cares? This is an excellent challenge. It's an excellent stressor. Most likely, this will be the hardest aspect of your injury. For some, it will do them in, and they will never return the same. And they won't ever be better. Not so for you. This is where you will learn about yourself. This is where you will learn how to quiet your mind and deal with the mental demons. You will learn how to exhale out the negative thoughts. You will learn how to replace those thoughts with proactive, positive thoughts. These thoughts will train and condition your Mindset each day. It will direct your focus and compel you to move forward. Ultimately you will learn how to take adversity and rise above it. You will learn how to fight and struggle and win no matter what stands before you. This lesson is so valuable, it's hard to think of others that matter as much. Setbacks, injuries, injustices, and pain in general are true gifts.

CHAPTER 45

RECOVERY - WAY OF INCHES

Last one. Remember. It's not how hard you can train. It's how hard you can train, recover fully, and train hard again, every day. Process is king. Let's look at what you're doing currently for your Recovery Block. And then let's improve it. Here's the test. Be honest with the assessment. It's only up from here.

RECOVERY

Injuries

- 10 Points: No major injuries for the year and missed no reps in games and practice.
- 8 Points: Hurt but missed no reps in games.
- 6 Points: Missed 20 percent of the games and practice reps.
- 4 Points: Missed 40 percent of game and practice reps.
- 0 Points: Missed more than half of the season.

POINTS: _____

Resting and Sleep Process

- 10 Points: You have a process to perfect performance and adhere to it always.
- 8 Points: You mostly have a process and adhere to it.
- 6 Points: You sometimes have a process and adhere to it.
- 4 Points: You rarely have a process and adhere to it.
- 0 Points: All else.

POINTS: _____

Treatments

- 10 Points: You have a process to perfect performance and adhere to it always.
- 8 Points: You mostly have a process and adhere to it.
- 6 Points: You sometimes have a process and adhere to it.
- 4 Points: You rarely have a process and adhere to it.
- 0 Points: All else.

POINTS: _____

Breathing and Meditation

- 10 Points: You have a process to perfect performance and adhere to it always.
- 8 Points: You mostly have a process and adhere to it.
- 6 Points: You sometimes have a process and adhere to it.
- 4 Points: You rarely have a process and adhere to it.
- 0 Points: All else.

POINTS: _____

Traveling

- 10 Points: You have a process to perfect performance and adhere to it always.
- 8 Points: You mostly have a process and adhere to it.
- 6 Points: You sometimes have a process and adhere to it.
- 4 Points: You rarely have a process and adhere to it.
- 0 Points: All else.

POINTS: _____

Kaizen

- 10 Points: You have a process for improving and adhere to it without fail.
- 8 Points: You mostly have a process and adhere to it.
- 5 Points: You occasionally have a process and adhere to it.
- 0 Points: All else.

POINTS: _____

Recovery Mentor

- 10 Points: You have one and connect weekly.
- 8 Points: You have one and connect monthly.
- 5 Points: You have one and connect quarterly.
- 0 Points: All else.

POINTS: _____

How effectively are you working with a Recovery accountability ally (or allies)?

- 10 Points: You and your ally review your results weekly, enforce a "carrot/stick," and adjust.
- 7 Points: You and your ally review your results monthly and sometimes enforce "carrot/stick."
- 4 Points: You and your ally review your results quarterly.
- 0 Points: All else.

POINTS: _____

You know your number one Recovery Strength (Competitive Advantage):

- 10 points. Otherwise: 0 points.

POINTS: _____

You know your number one Recovery Weakness (Weak Link):

- 10 points. Otherwise: 0 points.

POINTS: _____

You know your number one Recovery Opportunity (Target):

- 10 points. Otherwise: 0 points.

POINTS: _____

You know your number one Recovery Threat (Enemy):

- 10 points. Otherwise: 0 points.

POINTS: _____

TOTAL POINTS: _____

OVERALL AVERAGE (TOTAL POINTS /12) _____

Everything hinges on your Mindset Block. Do you have the Mindset to get better (Kaizen) in all areas as an athlete? As a person? If so, then the Recovery Block is as critical as any other Block. Ask yourself reflective questions at the end of each quarter:

- Do I have a plan for Recovery? How well do I implement it?
- What have been my habits for the last three months? What are two things I must do over the next three months to improve the Recovery Block?
- What are my obstacles? What are my solutions?
- Enjoyment is higher with a Teammate. Who will be on my side and help us advance together?

SWOT analysis. This time, apply your SWOT analysis to the Recovery Block. Be sure to prioritize and identify your Competitive Advantage and your Weak Link. You must advance in these areas to optimize your performance. Write out your process goals and habits for the next quarter. What is your number one Target for this quarter? Share with your Recovery accountability ally. Devise your carrot and stick for your check-ins. Bring on a mentor as well. I can't imagine a scenario where you work this diligently and don't advance. It's impossible. You'll continue to crush it. If you can't figure it out at all, then when in doubt, perfect your sleep habits.

- Strength:
  - List them all.
  - What are your top three?
  - What is your number one Strength (Competitive Advantage)?
- Weaknesses:
  - List them all.
  - What are your top three?
  - What is your number one Weakness (Weak Link)?
- Opportunities:
  - List them all.
  - What are your top three?
  - What is your number one Opportunity (Target)?
- Threats:
  - List them all.
  - What are your top three?
  - What is your number one Threat (Enemy)?

Recovery Way of Inches

Years ago, Duncan Sailors put out a book for tracking your training, aptly titled *Training Log*. It was a very simple book in a simple format. And it was quite useful. After all, we improve what we measure. One component of his *Training Log* was the Recovery Factor. If you can find it on-line it is worth the time and money.

Our inputs matter for any endeavor. Your recovery is no different. Now numbers don't lie, but they don't tell the entire story either. The trend of the numbers or data is more important than the data itself. And more important than the trend is the outcomes relative to the trend. And finally, most important is your adjustments to the outcomes. For example, you note that you average 8 hours of sleep a night, but you still feel sluggish on Friday nights before your game. Consequently, you start getting 9 hours of sleep on Thursday nights. And you notice you're no longer sluggish. As you continue to hunt for weaknesses, note what they are and fix them immediately. The following are a few reflective questions that will help guide you with your assessments:

- Sleep: How much do you need to feel optimal? What about the quality of your sleep?
- Nutrition: What's going into your mouth? Do you need more calories so you can recover?
- How banged up is your body?
- What recovery actions help most? Do you need to see a trainer and get worked on? Or is foam rolling all you need right now?

Once you have that data, then comes the most crucial step. Take the necessary actions to optimize your performance in the future! That's the whole point. Win. Win the day. Win the game. Now you know. Then write it down and do it.

Scan the following QR code or visit: https://athlete-builder.com to access and download the assessment in this chapter and other resources (free nutrition resources and free workout programs).

CHAPTER 46

THE WAY OF INCHES - ANNUAL PLAN

N ow is where the rubber meets the road. Time to work. I love the planning days and sessions. I'm always left with hope. I have a better plan of where I'm going, and I have high hopes of getting there. I also finish this exercise with renewed vigor and energy. It's great to feel this way with the Annual Plan and the Quarterly Plan. The feeling lasts about two days unfortunately. So, here's the "hack." In your daily and weekly plans, spend one to three minutes each morning looking over your long-term plans. If you remind yourself and rejuvenate yourself daily, then the feeling lasts. You very rarely wake each morning running out the door to attack the world and your endeavors. Energy simply doesn't arrive on your doorstep waiting for you. You must create it daily. Relentlessly.

- When do you conduct your Annual Review?
  - My business operates on a normal calendar year, so it's easy for me to have this review at the end of the year in December. That's an easy way for you to operate as well.
  - Here's something more effective: What's your sport season? If it's football, then it ends around Thanksgiving in high school. In college, it ends some time in December for most and a few in January. Pros end in January and February. The best time to have your annual review would be

two weeks after your season ends. Then you can assess and prepare for the upcoming "year" of your season.
  ° Get as much input from as many Teammates as possible. This includes your specific teammates, coaches, accountability allies, mentors, trainers, family, etc.

Inches Annual Review Process

- Block out days and times to work on your Annual Review. I lock myself in a cabin in Brown County, Indiana. Cell service is adequate. No one knows me there. And ultimately, it's quiet. I usually hike for a couple of hours each morning to clear my head. I work the entire rest of the day for the next two to three days. But that's for a full business with different components, a staff, etc. For you to do this on your own, give yourself one full morning (7:30–11:30) to do this. Your Quarterly Plan is done four times a year. One of those times coincides with your Annual Plan. Of course, that occasion will require more time and work. Make it fun; go somewhere secluded where you can reflect and get after it. The process will change over time, but the core structure will remain the same.
- Input important dates:
  ° Put in the obvious ones: holidays, vacations, birthdays, etc.
  ° Put in the critical ones: games, practices, spring season, playoffs, etc. These are the performance dates. Being great in your own workouts is nice. Practices, too. . . nice. Games are what matter. Results are why we do this and work this hard. No one is great on game day without being Relentless in practice. At the same time, no one cares what you "benched in high school" or do in practice. Performance matters now. "You are what the scoreboard says you are," said Bill Parcels.
- Take the Assessment Test. Note and track your score.

- Conduct your Annual Review. Keep track of your notes as well.

Annual Review

Mindset

This part of your assessment only applies to the Mindset Block.

- What were your wins in the prior year? List them all. Each one matters. Prioritize and rank them.
- What were your losses in the prior year? List them all. Each one matters here as well. Prioritize and rank them.
- What lessons did you learn from your wins and losses? Habits form from lessons. You must recognize the pattern in the lessons. Then you can adjust your habits. Changing your habits leads to new patterns and results. This is what you want for the next year. Everyone has already started to forget what you, your team, and everyone else did last season. You must not. Get a head start on the competition and move ahead of the pack.
- What Mindset habits helped you the most last year? Which hurt you the most? What must you do this year to improve?
- What are your reasons to be grateful? Remember, somewhere there's a child at St. Jude's Children's Hospital hoping he sees some athlete or celebrity once before he or she dies. And ultimately, we are playing a game or trying to play one for a living. Jesus put you here to maximize your talents and abilities in His honor. Be grateful and humble.
- What other notes do you have on the season/year? Great memories? Moments? Relationships? What stood out?

Knowledge

Conduct the same approach here. But apply it solely to the Knowledge side.

- What were your wins? What did you learn about your sport?
- What were your losses? What did you not learn about your sport? What must you still learn? This is your target for next year.
- What are your reasons to be grateful?
- What other notes do you have about the Knowledge Block?

Teammates

Conduct the same approach here. But apply it solely to the Teammate side.

- What were your wins? Which relationships had the most impact? Which ones helped you?
- What were your losses? Which relationships were a struggle for you? Which hurt your results?
- What must you do this year to improve the weak relationships and keep the strong ones?
- Which relationships must you let go? This is important.
- What are your reasons to be grateful?
- What other notes do you have on the Teammate Block?

Training

Conduct the same approach here. But apply it solely to the Training Block.

- What were your wins? What were your biggest improvements? What do you do very well? You must continue to improve your strengths next year.
- What were your losses? What don't you do very well? You will target your weaknesses next year.
- What lessons did you learn? What is holding you back?
- What are your reasons to be grateful?
- What other notes do you have on the Training Block?

Nutrition

Conduct the same approach here. But apply it solely to the Nutrition Block.

- What were your wins? What did you do well?
- What were your losses? What Nutrition habit hurt you the most?
- What lessons did you learn? What must you still learn?
- What are your reasons to be grateful?
- What other notes do you have on the Nutrition Block?

Recovery

Conduct the same approach here. But apply it solely to the Recovery Block.

- What were your wins? What helped you recover consistently?
- What were your losses? Any injuries or nagging ailments?

- What lessons did you learn? What must you add to your Recovery routine?
- What are your reasons to be grateful?
- What other notes do you have on the Recovery Block?

Next, where are we going next year and beyond? Take some time. Think. Go for a walk. Think some more. Refine your thoughts. And think some more! Develop answers to the following questions:

- Who must you become to achieve, to win, and to accomplish your goals? What does that look like?
- What are your Core Values? What do you stand for?
- What is your ultimate path? What does that look like one year, three years, and longer down the road?
- What is your mission this year? What is the main thing this year? Write this down. Put it on Post-it notes in your bathroom. Put it as your screensaver on all electronics.
- What is the mission for your team? Typically, the coaches provide that. So, take what they give you and add your "Inches Premium." What's that mean? It means that whatever the coach asks of the team, you add 10–30 percent minimum on top of that. And you and your unit work under that Mindset and directive.
- What is the mission for your unit? Again, typically your position coach will have a directive. It may be that the back line of defense on your soccer team commits to allowing no more than ten shots on goal per game. You add the "Inches Premium" and you make it harder by 10–30 percent. That means your unit can only allow seven to nine shots on goal per game.
- What is your mission for yourself personally? This one is challenging and critical. It will define your standard of excellence in the next year and season. Example: It's October 24, 2022 right now as I'm writing this. On September 30, 2021, I decided to add cold therapy to my regimen for daily improvement. I committed

that I would add in cold showers every time I showered over the next year. I started with a simple fifteen-second adaptation approach the first time. Well, now it's almost thirteen months later. I don't miss. Whenever I shower (home, vacation, holidays, a hotel, a relative's house), I do three to five minutes of cold showers. In addition, I've added ice baths for four to six minutes multiple times per week, in all seasons, outside. My mission was to become healthier once I decided to retire from competing in powerlifting and strongman. This was part of it. I did it. And I'm still doing it. It never ends. Kaizen is a Core Value.

- What is your mantra for the next year? Is there a theme? Halfway into my son Jack's second season of college football, I asked him what the coach wanted of his play. Jack said that coach wanted him to be very physical (duh, he's a linebacker) and be the first one to the correct spot on the field. So, I said, "Simple. Your mantra is 'fast and physical.'" What's your mantra for the next season?

- How will you feel in twelve months once you've reached these milestones? Be specific. Write it down. See how accurate you are. What will it mean for you to get to that level?

- Here's an important step: What obstacles will get in your way? Prioritize them. Write out solutions. And execute Relentlessly in the next twelve months. Discipline. Plan all the way to the end.

- What are the necessary tools you'll need to execute? Do you need a personal coach? Different equipment? New routines? Get them. Buy them. Create them. Find them. Make it happen and move forward!

Good. That's your Annual Review. You have assessed your year and have ideas and goals for the next year. You will refine it more with the Quarterly Review. Then you will map out your targets and habits with the Monthly Review. It will be more specific with your weekly Review and the six critical Inch Targets. The daily review is "game day." Let's see how you compete every day and what you learn. You win your year by winning every day.

CHAPTER 47

THE WAY OF INCHES - QUARTERLY PLAN

Like the Annual Plan, you'll need some time away from people and distractions. Then you can dial in and focus on yourself and your journey. You'll need either a morning or afternoon to do this. Of course, your plan for the first quarter will coincide with your Annual Plan preparations. Naturally, you'll need more time to complete your Annual Plan and your first Quarterly Plan together.

- Take the Assessment Test again. Keep track of your scores in Inch Blocks.
- Then revisit your "7 Levels of Why." This is performance-related for you and your sport.
- Where are you going from now until the end of time? I refer to this as "climbing your mountain." This thought encompasses your life mission. If that's too far off in the distance to understand, then where must you go in the next three months?
- Then ask yourself "Why?" Why are you doing this? Then "Why?" again. Then "Why?" again. And again and again and again. Eventually you'll come to the root reason. It's the fundamental, basic reason you're doing this. However, it's also very important to know each "Why" that you're doing things. They add up in a big way.

Let's say a new student athlete walks into my gym to meet with me. I say, "All right, kid, why are you here to train at Unbreakable Athletics?"

He answers, "To get better at soccer."

"Why?"

"So I can play varsity as a sophomore."

I ask him again: "Why?"

"So I can be the best on the team by my senior year."

"Why?"

"So I can earn a college scholarship."

"Why?"

"So my parents don't have to pay for school, and I don't have to get loans."

One more time: "Why?"

"Because we don't have a lot of money. And I'm only the second person in my family to go to college. And I want to become an engineer and build things one day."

See that? That's his "Why." He wants a certain lifestyle in the future while helping his family not pay for college. This is his approach to creating it and taking control of it. It only took six "Whys" to get there. Sometimes it's two or three "Whys." Other times it's eight to ten. But this is his main "Why." Find yours and post it everywhere as a reminder.

Here is what is also cool. More importantly, it is more empowering. He has his main "Why" (free college to be an engineer). He also has other "Whys" that he can stack: play as a sophomore, best as a senior, alleviating the burden on his parents. I'm assuming he may have even more: He feels great about himself because he's the best (ego); it proves to himself he could do it; his friends said he couldn't do it; no one has done it from his school before; etc., etc. And the list goes on and on. The seemingly lesser "Whys" are powerful too.

Harness all the power together. Keep your main "Why" at the top, but don't forget all the other "Whys" required to build up to it. Keep those in mind too. Post the "Whys" where you'll see them repeatedly: phone, tablet, laptop, sticky notes on your mirror, on your fridge, in your car, above your bed. Harness that power and use it to create tremendous action and momentum.

- If this is your first time, then this next question won't work. Otherwise, it will. What has changed any of your "Whys" since the last quarter? Are there any new ones? Are you getting rid of any prior "Whys"? Make a new list every quarter if there are updates.
- Other than yourself, for whom else in your life do you want to do this? Family or friends? Teammates or coworkers? Your faith? If your "Why" is greater than you and your goals, then it becomes even more powerful and influential.
- How urgent is your "Why" this quarter? If it's the quarter before the season starts, it's more urgent. If it's the quarter before your last season, it is supremely more urgent.

Next, we will progress through the six different Inch Blocks. We will explore through more reflective questions to gain insights. Then we will progress through the process. This is the *Inches 365* process. It's the systematic path for achieving your highest levels and results.

Take notes here. Really. Pay attention. When athletes walk into my gym to improve, we never throw everything at them right away. We don't change their Nutrition, their Recovery, their Training, etc. all at once. It's overwhelming. It's not sustainable. Everyone, and I mean everyone, quits if we do that. The only group that can get away with a full twenty-four-hour-a-day life change is the military. The military gets away with it because you're locked in for four years and can't quit. We change one habit at a time until it's set and solid. Then we do another and another until you've maxed out and can't improve (never).

What does this mean for you? When you start making changes, don't overload yourself and make too many changes at once! You'll quit. You'll quit. You'll quit. Make one change in each area for two to three weeks and see how you do. Then, and only then, evolve further and change another habit to improve. After a while, you will ingrain some habits, and they are set. Then it will be time to take another step forward. For example, I've trained a minimum of four times a week for ten years. That's not a challenging thing for me anymore. I just do it.

Go through the questions below. Do your homework and assessments. And pick some things to address. What you'll see below is the format for when you're clicking on all cylinders. Work up to it. I didn't deadlift 600 lb. the first day. It took me eight years from age thirty-seven to forty-five. Imagine if I lifted and trained from fourteen on, I can't even imagine.

The word is *sustainable*. Create a lifestyle of evolving that is sustainable. Look one, three, five, ten, twenty years down the road and where you're going. And then attack every day.

Mindset

- Start with the 7 Levels of Why and complete that thoroughly.
- Score yourself in relation to the 6 Core Values (Integrity, Discipline, Kaizen, Teamwork, Enjoyment, Sisu). Where would you put yourself in relation to the 6 Core Values? Score yourself from 1 (terrible and should quit the sport) to 10 (Hall-of-Fame-level "Statue").
- Where would you put yourself in relation to our mantra, "Relentless"? (Score from 1 to 10.)
- How did you do overall in the last quarter? Score yourself against what your plans and processes were last quarter. Also score yourself against your unit on your team, your team overall, and other teams in the conference and league. (Score from 1 to 10.)
- Are you doing your best (Integrity)? (Score from 1 to 10.)
- Are you enjoying the game and process enough? This means that you might not love the pain of the process, but you do love the results. And that will carry you, and that's okay (Enjoyment). (Score from 1 to 10.)
- How resilient are you (Sisu)? (Score from 1 to 10.)

- Do you have a process for improving? How well are you adhering to it (Discipline)? (Score from 1 to 10.)
- What limiting beliefs and fears are holding you back (Kaizen)? This is a negative score here if you are being held back. However, if you have fears and a process to address them, then it is a positive score as long as you keep moving forward through your fears consistently. (Score from −10 to +10.)

Mindset Way of Inches

You'll need to conduct a SWOT Analysis. It's a business term that is everywhere.

Strengths: List all your strengths. Then prioritize your top three. What is your top, main strength? Your number one Strength? This is your Competitive Advantage. This is the one thing that you are best at. You want to make sure this thing becomes the one thing you are better at doing than anyone else in the world at doing. Example: Wal-Mart is the best at being the lowest-cost provider of retail goods. Amazon is the best at getting goods delivered to people's homes. Develop things that you are best at, and you can win. And it's more fun doing things that you're great at.

Weaknesses: List all your weaknesses. Then prioritize your main three weaknesses that you must improve at once. Then, what is the biggest weakness holding you back? Your number one weakness? That is your limiting factor, your Weak Link. It's your weak link in the chain, and a chain is only as strong as its weakest link. Improve your limiting factor, and you must be better at once.

Opportunities: List the three main (Mindset) opportunities you have in the next quarter. As an example, maybe it's the first quarter after the football season ends. You may be lacking confidence. Now your opportunity becomes the chance to become secure and confident in your abilities. If you put in the time, hours, and preparation in all areas, then your confidence must improve. You must play better after all that work.

What is the most important Mindset opportunity you have? This is your number one target.

Threats: List your Mindset threats here. This is the component that can really hurt you. Going back to the last example, if your confidence is a problem, then you'll "play slow," play badly, and most likely move down the depth chart. Even more important, playing slow means you're creating less force as an athlete. (Force = Mass × Acceleration. Slowing down = Less Force.) Creating less force in sport leads to consistent injuries. You must be aware of the threats but never dwell on them. You must continue to spend your time improving your strengths and weaknesses. This will decrease and mitigate your threats. Focus there mentally and watch your threats simply fade away.

Next, set two or three process goals and habits in this area. Make sure one habit in the next quarter advances your best strength, your competitive advantage. Set one habit to bring up your biggest weakness, your limiting factor. Then add one more habit in anything you want to improve. Critical: Of your three new habits, what is your *one* habit that you must do? This is your number one target, so if you hit this target, then the other targets won't be as important or even necessary.

Seek out help. Who is your Accountability Ally or Mentor in this area? Discuss your plans and make any changes if necessary. Then establish your rewards/punishments (carrot/stick) for not meeting your standards and habits. Check in weekly. Schedule it. Get feedback from your ally, mentor, or both and adjust each week. This will be huge! Even the best of all time, like Kobe Bryant and Michael Jordan, had mentors and help from those that came before them. It's critical. Take their knowledge and run. It makes life and progress easier and faster.

Lastly, track your habits and results week to week, month to month, and all quarter long. Improving will be easy at that point. Apply the process Relentlessly, and each iteration will be better than the last. This is the way, Inches 365.

Knowledge

Here we go again. Ask yourself a series of reflective questions and gauge your progress over the last quarter.

- What's your level of Knowledge of the playbook? More importantly, what is your level of Knowledge for playing your position at the highest level? (Score from 1 to 10.)
- What's your level of Knowledge of the other positions on your team so you can lead them on the field? What is your level of Knowledge of the players and how they work so you can motivate and get the most out of them as well? (Score from 1 to 10.)
- What's your level of Knowledge of the teams on your schedule? Personnel, strengths, weaknesses, and tendencies? (Score from 1 to 10.)
- What's your level of life-skill Knowledge? (Score from 1 to 10.)

Knowledge Way of Inches

This time, apply your SWOT analysis to the Knowledge component, not Mindset. Be sure to prioritize and identify your Competitive Advantage and your Weak Link. You must advance in these areas to optimize your performance. Write out your process goals and habits for the next quarter. What is your number one target for this quarter? Share with your Knowledge accountability ally or mentor. (Remember, you may need only one ally or mentor, or more than one.) Devise your carrot and stick for your check-ins. I can't imagine a scenario where you work this diligently and don't advance. Improving your strengths and weaknesses is how you hit your targets and minimize your threats. Keep at it.

- Strengths: Top Three Knowledge Strengths?

- ○ Number one Strength, Competitive Advantage?
- ○ Number one Habit to work on next quarter to advance your competitive advantage?
- Weaknesses: Top Three Knowledge Weaknesses?
  - ○ Number one Weakness, Weak Link?
  - ○ Number one Habit to work on next quarter to improve your weak link?
- Opportunities: Top Three Knowledge Opportunities?
  - ○ Number one Opportunity, or Target?
- Threats: Top Three Knowledge Threats?
  - ○ Number one Threat?
- Mentor or Ally: Who is it? What are the carrots and sticks for hitting weekly goals?

Teammates

How are you at leading and helping others (Teamwork)? Can you and are you helping anyone with their own Mindset, Knowledge, Training, Nutrition, and Recovery areas? You don't have to lead the entire team at first. Find one person and help him or her improve. Start there and expand.

Do you want to see magic happen? Imagine you're a linebacker and the entire linebacking unit is unified and attacking these six areas Relentlessly. What does that look like? It looks like a stifling defense, like the 1985 Chicago Bears, who set every defense record imaginable on their way to a one-loss season and smashing the New England Patriots in the Super Bowl. A half dozen of those guys ended up in the Hall of Fame. They were great Teammates.

- Do you help lead and hold others accountable? (Score from 1 to 10.)
- How would you score your ability to collaborate with the coaches and support staff? (Score from 1 to 10.)

- How would you score your ability to work with your other professional and personal team? (Score from 1 to 10.)
- Do you make others better? Show appreciation? Elevate the world around you? (Score from 1 to 10.)

Teammates Way of Inches

Again, conduct your SWOT analysis. Prioritize and identify the keys in your Strengths, Weaknesses, Opportunities, and Threats. Locate your Competitive Advantage and Weak Link. Plan to improve both. Work with your accountability ally and mentor. Track and adjust. Be Relentless!

- Strengths: Top Three Teammate Strengths?
    - Number one Strength, Competitive Advantage?
    - Number one habit to work on next quarter to advance your competitive advantage?
- Weaknesses: Top Three Teammate Weaknesses?
    - Number one Weakness, Weak Link?
    - Number one Habit to work on next quarter to improve your weak link?
- Opportunities: Top Three Teammate Opportunities?
    - Number one Opportunity, or Target?
- Threats: Top Three Teammate Threats?
    - Number one Threat?
- Mentor or Ally: Who is it? What are the carrots and sticks for hitting weekly goals?

Training

Physically, where are you at? What can you do consistently? What's that look like?

- Physical strength? Where are you strong, weak compared to your-self last quarter and to your competitors? (Score from 1 to 10.)
- Speed and explosiveness? Same thing here. Where are you better and worse compared to your abilities and your competitors? (Score from 1 to 10.)
- What's your stamina like? Can you handle late game work and overtime? Are you in the best shape or in need of work? (Score from 1 to 10.)
- What about "bulletproofing your body"? For example, it's not overly necessary to have huge biceps in football. A strong back, core, and lower body would be higher priorities. That's all true until you get hit in the arm at a high rate of force by someone else's helmet. Then you're going to wish your arm were protected by a lot of huge muscle mass. Louie Simmons would say, "No weaknesses anywhere." And it's true. (Score from 1 to 10.)
- Physically, what's your body at overall? Are you on the bench? A starter? All-American? A Pro? All Pro? Are you at the Statue level? (Score from 1 to 10.)

Training Way of Inches

Do a thorough SWOT analysis here. This could take a minute. You might be a very strong squatter (Strength). But if your quads are huge and your hamstrings lag, this creates an imbalance here that could easily lead to injury (Weakness). The Opportunity is to bring up the lagging muscle group before the Threat of injury occurs. So, take your time. Be thorough. Set up a meeting with your strength coach. And then find data for comparison. In Ohio State's weight room, there is a board posted with the results of the prior year's combine numbers. It will have the top 10 percent and one standard deviation numbers. No one cares about the bottom two-thirds. So, they strive for the top. Get your numbers to match those, and now you're in the discussion.

Process here is king. It's also a huge challenge! Huge! Most high school and college coaches can't get you there. They can't. So many are not very good at all. It's true. They love all the cute little gadgets and data and numbers. They only prioritize speed and quickly forget that strength is a bigger base in the pyramid of the athlete. It's criminal. Embarrassing. Pathetic, really. Then there are those who are very good, but the funding is limited. The staff has an entire football team of a hundred kids. Then they could have other sports teams to work with too. There is limited time in the weight room. Too many kids and not enough resources. It's so hard. Finally at the top, there are those who are legit coaches and have the resources. Look out then. Those teams are going to destroy the competition.

What does this mean for you? You must get smart on your own. You must train extra on your own. You must figure it out, advocate for yourself. You must make it happen. No one is coming to save you. Mommy and Daddy can't "helicopter parent" your way to success.

Example: Your grip is weak because it's not trained. Then you will be a weaker tackler or ball receiver. Or your neck and traps are weak. Then you're more susceptible to concussions. If you have a weak core and back. . . then you are simply weak everywhere. You'll get injured for sure. What do I mean by weak core? Here's a test: Get in a plank hold and put 1× your bodyweight in sandbags along your back. Hold it for one full minute. So, if you weigh 250 lb., then load up 250 lb. of weight and see. (If you need a legit coach, I know a guy. ☺)

Now go through your SWOT analysis. Set your habits and goals. Find allies and mentors. Track your results and adjust. Your Weak Link will always be a moving target. You'll need to readjust often. Your Training is very important. This where it "takes a village" to get enough support to perfect your physical abilities. You'll need multiple sources help here.

- Strengths: Top Three Training Strengths?
  - Number one Strength, Competitive Advantage?
  - Number one Habit to work on next quarter to advance your competitive advantage?
- Weaknesses: Top Three Training Weaknesses?
  - Number one Weakness, Weak Link?
  - Number one Habit to work on next quarter to improve your weak link?
- Opportunities: Top Three Training Opportunities?
  - Number one Opportunity, or Target?
- Threats: Top Three Training Threats?
  - Number one Threat?
- Mentor or Ally: Who is it? What are the carrots and sticks for hitting weekly goals?

Nutrition

Two-thirds of your physical success is a result of your diet. For some, it's 60 percent. Others, it's 90 percent. A lot of athletes will tell you that the work of putting in the right food and amount of food is much harder than the training needed for success. Just ask around. Take Brian Shaw, 6′7″ and 440 lb. He would consume 14,000 calories a day (not a typo) to compete at World's Strongest Man. And he won more than most others on the planet. Then look at Michael Phelps. He's 6′5″ and lean, but he'd take in the same number of calories because he was burning that many calories each day swimming in the Olympics. It takes what it takes. (I can't imagine the amount of time spent on the toilet!)

- Can you eat to perform? (Score from 1 to 10.)
- What are your hydration habits? In-season? When it's hot and humid? Example: Ever see the football guys cramping early in the season when they play in the South, where it's hot? Yeah. . . not hydrated and prepared properly. They missed reps. Were in pain. Not effective. That was easily avoidable. (Score from 1 to 10.)
- Are you on top of your game with supplements? (Score from 1 to 10.)
- Are you training hard but not making gains? That will be a result of food and/or recovery. (Score from 1 to 10.)
- What about eating to perform on game day? How does your body react? Can you perfect it? (Score from 1 to 10.)
- What's your body fat? What's the best body fat percentage for you to be at your best in your sport? (Score from 1 to 10.)
- What about when you travel? What changes? What's your process? (Score from 1 to 10.)

Nutrition Way of Inches

Same drill here. Run through your SWOT analysis. Identify the keys, competitive advantages, and weak links. Prioritize the areas you want to improve. Make adjustments. Get help from allies and mentors. Make your plan and execute. Carrots and sticks. This will be a moving target too. Over the years, your body will change, as will your metabolism. Get some help here. You'll need it.

- Strengths: Top Three Nutrition Strengths?
  - Number one Strength, Competitive Advantage?
  - Number one Habit to work on next quarter to advance your competitive advantage?
- Weaknesses: Top Three Nutrition Weaknesses?
  - Number one Weakness, Weak Link?

- ◦ Number one Habit to work on next quarter to improve your weak link?
- Opportunities: Top Three Nutrition Opportunities?
  - ◦ Number one Opportunity, or Target?
- Threats: Top Three Nutrition Threats?
  - ◦ Number one Threat?
- Mentor or Ally: Who is it? What are the carrots and sticks for hitting weekly goals?

Recovery

Anyone can train hard for a day or two or even a week. But is it sustainable? Can you train hard on Monday and still smash it Tuesday? It's not how hard can you train. It's how hard can you train, then recover, and train hard again. That's the deal. Once you have your nutrition dialed in, then it's all about recovery. The following are questions for reflection. You may or may not already have experience with these recovery methods. If you do, assess as best you can the effectiveness of each technique. Then assess your frequency of applying the methods. On the flip side, if you haven't tried the following methods, then you should seek out your coach for instructions or contact us at Athlete Builder for guidance and coaching.

- What steps do you take to perfect your resting and recovery?
- What about healing and treatments? Are you consistent? Deliberate and effective?
- Ice baths and cold showers?
- Meditation and breathing?
- What needs to be different during the week, during camp, during the season, or after games?
- What about when you travel? Jet lag?
- What about when the weather is a significant factor? Playing in extreme weather adds to the stress a normal game puts on a player.

Recovery Way of Inches

Last one here. Take it seriously. It's why athletes go to steroids and performance enhancing drugs. They help with Recovery. Here's the thing. If you're diligent and Relentless in applying the tools for Recovery, then it will take you to about 97–98 percent of your recovery potential. The extra "juice" only adds a few percent. So why bother? You'll get caught and kicked out of the league. And your body will be wrecked for using it. So, don't! But do everything else.

Conduct your SWOT analysis and run yourself through the process. Keep prioritizing and executing. Get help from allies and mentors. Keep pushing up your competitive advantages and raise your weakest links. It'll be awesome.

- Strengths: Top Three Recovery Strengths?
  - Number one Strength, Competitive Advantage?
  - Number one Habit to work on next quarter to advance your competitive advantage?
- Weaknesses: Top Three Recovery Weaknesses?
  - Number one Weakness, Weak Link?
  - Number one Habit to work on next quarter to improve your weak link?
- Opportunities: Top Three Recovery Opportunities?
  - Number one Opportunity, or Target?
- Threats: Top Three Recovery Threats?
  - Number one Threat?
- Mentor or Ally: Who is it? What are the carrots and sticks for hitting weekly goals?

Remember what you read at the beginning of this section. Sustainability is key. Consistent progress is much more valuable than a huge effort done rarely. It's easy to get overwhelmed. It's also easy not to get overwhelmed. How? Only do the number one habits you must do.

Don't worry about adding five or six or more habits. Just do the number one habits for your strengths and weaknesses. Be diligent daily. It will add Inches and push you up your mountain.

CHAPTER 48

THE WAY OF INCHES - MONTHLY PLAN

The first month in the Monthly Plan is simply scheduling out what you decided to do in your Quarterly Plan. The assessment and questions are similar and shorter as well. You must still schedule a date and time to do this. I like to do it on the last Friday of the month. That way, next month I can hit the ground running. I usually do the work over lunch that day and have my calendar blocked off for that purpose.

First take ten to fifteen minutes and start off by asking yourself the basics:

- What wins did you have last month in the six key areas (Mindset, Knowledge, Teammates, Training, Nutrition, and Recovery)?
- What losses did you have?
- What reasons do you have to be grateful?
- What lessons did you learn?
- Were there any obstacles? If so, what were the solutions?
- Was your mantra effective last month? What is it next month?

Then you'll need to do some reminder work. Look over your notes of what your plans are for the year and this quarter specifically. If you consistently remind and engage yourself with your targets, it'll help generate clarity and energy. Spend ten to fifteen minutes here and make any necessary adjustments.

Spend the last thirty minutes of your hour breaking down the six Inches 365 Blocks. It's five minutes per Block:

Mindset: What are your one to two process goals for the next month? What are your carrot and stick? What does your accountability ally and/or mentor have to say?

Knowledge: What are your one to two process goals for the next month? What are your carrot and stick? What does your accountability ally and/or mentor have to say?

Teammates: What are your one to two process goals for the next month? What are your carrot and stick? What does your accountability ally and/or mentor have to say?

Training: What are your one to two process goals for the next month? What are your carrot and stick? What does your accountability ally and/or mentor have to say?

Nutrition: What are your one to two process goals for the next month? What are your carrot and stick? What does your accountability ally and/or mentor have to say?

Recovery: What are your one to two process goals for the next month? What are your carrot and stick? What does your accountability ally and/or mentor have to say?

That's it. Then you're good to go. Added tips: One month, do this work alongside one of your Teammates. Then you both can improve. Another month, do this work alongside a mentor. Then you can receive additional insights. One month, ask a coach to meet with you briefly to discuss the topics he coaches. It could be your position coach or your strength coach. One month, meet with a nutrition expert for help. One month, schedule a consultation and time with me or my team and see how quickly we can advance you. You don't know what you don't know.

CHAPTER 49

THE WAY OF INCHES - WEEKLY PLAN

M y wife and I call it "getting our life in order." We do this every Sunday afternoon, usually after family dinner. We have a late breakfast after church. Then family dinner is about 3:30–4:00. Afterward we'll spend some time planning out our week and getting everything lined up so we can execute. It doesn't take long.

We start with three questions:

- What were the wins and losses last week?
- What are the reasons to be grateful?
- What obstacles and solutions presented themselves? What did you learn?

Then we go through the reminders:

- What are your main targets for the year, this quarter, and this month specifically?
- What is your mantra this month and this week specifically?

Then we schedule our habits. As you know, there are six Inches 365 Blocks. Each Block has a task every day. Here is an example of the work I did on my Mindset Blocks. A couple years ago, I wanted to spend more time doing devotional work. Ideally, I'd do this every day like my wife always does. So, I found an app I liked to use, and I decided I'd add this habit to my morning routine. The minimum number of times each week I wanted to do this was four. Five times was my main goal. My stretch goal was seven times each week. Each time I spent time on devotional work, I'd mark it in my planner. Then, at the end of the week, I'd see how I did.

Let's look at the Nutrition Block as an example for you. Maybe one of your targets is to improve your protein intake for your performance. The minimum goal would be to track how much protein you consume daily. (Remember, we improve what we measure.) And let's assume your target is one gram of protein for every pound of body weight. So, if you weigh two hundred pounds, then you need two hundred grams of daily protein. Your main goal might be to get this in five times a week. And your stretch goal would be seven times a week. After a while, you always track your protein. And you're hitting your numbers seven times a week because you plan your meals and it's now easy. Good job! So, then you add in your next habit of taking your creatine and supplements. For this, I put my pill container of supplements and creatine right by my toothbrush. Each morning, I brush my teeth and take my supplements. I "stack" my new habit (supplements) with one habit I have done for decades (brushing my teeth). For three years, I used a weekly pill container. Recently, I got rid of that one and bought one that is filled monthly. Now I must fill it only once per month. It's still right by my toothbrush. Now I've been doing it daily for a month and it's easier.

Last thing we do is schedule out our week. Put in your time constraints (school, work, practice, training, meal prep, events, etc.). Then schedule when you'll execute your habits for the six Inch Blocks. Schedule in when you'll talk with your allies and mentors. With the time remaining, do whatever you like next week. That's it. You're good to go.

CHAPTER 50

THE WAY OF INCHES - DAILY PLAN

The days are long, but the years are short. At this point, most of your week is blocked off and scheduled. Not it's time to execute deliberately. Block out ten minutes at the beginning and end of each day. We need to go over your morning and evening routine.

Morning Routine

- Get up early and weigh in.
- Take in your water and supplements.
- If you have time, take a short walk to clear your head. Pray and/or meditate. Instill your mantra for the day. No time for the walk? Sit quietly and get your head right.
- If you can, shower up and add in a cold shower or ice bath if this aligns with your habits. If you're not there yet, it's cool. Just clean up and get ready to go.
- Look over your schedule and refine your notes. Be very mindful of what your Mindset must be as you approach each meeting, event, or task.

This part is very important. You have six tasks today. They are your Inches 365 tasks. There is one each for the six Blocks (Mindset, Knowledge, Teammates, Training, Nutrition, and Recovery).

You must complete the six tasks today. The six tasks are the priority. Get this done. This is how you win. Everything else helps quite a bit. But the six tasks matter the most and help the most. Just do it.

- Identify any major targets, obstacles or stressors and solutions. Be very deliberate here. These will be the events to execute well.
- Note a reason to be grateful and something to look forward to doing.
- Solidify your mantra. Attack your day.

Now your day is over. How did you do? Take a moment to reflect and wind down. Make notes in your planner or journal. Sometimes I'll do this before I even get home. I'll conduct all my assessments and leave it at work. Then when I'm home, I focus solely on my family and de-stressing.

Evening Routine

- What were the major wins, losses, and lessons learned in the six Inch Blocks? What other wins, losses, and lessons were learned as well?
- Write down any necessary notes for your weekly assessment this coming Friday.
- Quit your electronics and TV thirty to sixty minutes prior to going to bed.
- Read, mediate, and/or pray. What can you be grateful about that day?
- Decrease your fluid intake so you're not up all night.
- Keep your room as cold as tolerable and put on some white noise like a fan.

- Set your alarm and room up for the next morning. In most everything, your environment is key. Set your environment up for success.

That's it. Tomorrow is a new day to attack. Be Relentless.

About the Author

Jim Beebe is the Founder and Head Coach of Unbreakable Athletics Academy in Plainfield, IN, where he has coached over 400 student athletes, with more than 10% advancing to play college sports, including many at the Division I level. He has also coached over 1,000 adults in CrossFit, strength training, and nutrition. Jim is a seasoned competitor in Strongman, Powerlifting, CrossFit, Olympic Lifting, and obstacle course races, with certifications in Powerlifting, CrossFit, and Strongman. A Purdue University graduate with a BS and MS in Finance, he also hosts the Athlete Builder podcast and travels extensively for public speaking and coaching. As the Founder and Head Coach of Athlete Builder, an online coaching service, Jim aims to work with 20,000 college athletes and produce two national title winners by 2028, using a systematic approach that develops both the minds and bodies of athletes. Jim and his wife, Jen, have 6 children together: Kate, Jack, Lauren, Maddie, Sam, and Madi.

Printed in the USA
CPSIA information can be obtained
at www.ICGtesting.com
CBHW031907281024
16539CB00002B/2